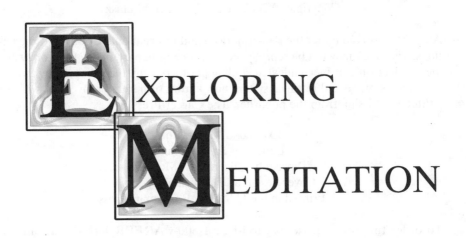

EXPLORING MEDITATION

Master the Ancient Art of
Relaxation and Enlightenment

By

Dr. Susan G. Shumsky

NEW PAGE BOOKS
A division of The Career Press, Inc.
Franklin Lakes, NJ

EXPLORING MEDITATION
Edited by Tracy Collins
Typeset by Eileen Dow Munson
Cover design by The Visual Group
Printed in the U.S.A. by Book-mart Press

To order this title, please call toll-free 1-800-CAREER-1 (NJ and Canada: 201-848-0310) to order using VISA or MasterCard, or for further information on books from Career Press.

Divine Revelation is a service mark registered with the United States Patent Office.

 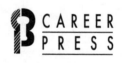

The Career Press, Inc., 3 Tice Road, PO Box 687,
Franklin Lakes, NJ 07417
www.careerpress.com
www.newpagebooks.com

Library of Congress Cataloging-in-Publication Data

Shumsky, Dr. Susan G.
   Exploring meditation ; master the ancient art of relaxation and enlightenment / by Susan Shumsky.
      p. cm.
   Includes bibliographical references and index.
   ISBN 1-56414-562-X (pbk.)
   1. Meditation--Hinduism. 2. Yoga. 3. Spiritual life--Hinduism. I. Title

BL1238.32 .s58 2001
294.5'435--dc21

2001044285

All the testimonials in this book are real, but some names, occupations, or places of residence have been changed.

Exploring Meditation can familiarize you with the complex field of meditation, spiritual development, and Yoga, but in no way claims to fully teach the techniques described. Therefore, personal instruction is recommended. *Exploring Meditation* is not an independent guide for self-healing. Susan Shumsky is not a medical doctor and does not diagnose diseases or prescribe treatments. No medical claims are implied about any methods, exercises, or postures suggested in this book, even if specific "benefits" or "healing" of diseases or conditions are mentioned. The methods and suggestions in this book should be followed only under guidance and supervision of a medical doctor or psychiatrist. Susan Shumsky, her agents, assigns, licensees, and authorized representatives, as well as Divine Revelation, Teaching of Intuitional Metaphysics, and Career Press, make no claim or obligation and take no legal responsibility for the effectiveness, results, or benefits of reading this book, of using the methods described, or of contacting anyone listed in this book or at *www.divinerevelation.org*; deny all liability for any injuries or damages that you may incur; and are to be held harmless against any claim, liability, loss or damage caused by or arising from following any suggestions made in this book or from contacting anyone listed in this book or at *www.divinerevelation.org*.

This book is dedicated to
seekers of truth everywhere.
If you could only see
how precious you truly are,
you would realize that
what you are seeking is
what you already are.

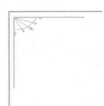

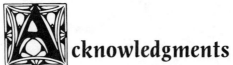
Acknowledgments

I give gratitude to my beautiful inner teachers, who are guiding me night and day with tireless dedication and devotion. Your love and support bring this wisdom to the world.

I am deeply grateful to Jeff Herman and Deborah Adams for your true friendship, compassion, spirit, and undaunted perseverance, even through the greatest challenges. I especially thank you for not giving up on me. I thank Mike Lewis for believing in this book and Stacey Farkas and Tracey Collins for bringing it to completion.

I give gratitude to all those who brought these beautiful teachings to me. I thank Maharishi Mahesh Yogi, first and foremost, for opening my mind to higher states of consciousness and for his Vedic wisdom. My gratitude goes to Dr. Peter Victor Meyer, Dr. Ann Meyer Makeever, Rich Bell, and Joanna Cherry for bringing me the precious knowledge of Divine Revelation. I thank Ved Prakash for his contributions to this work.

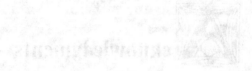

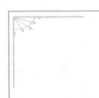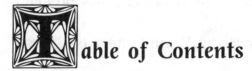

Table of Contents

Part III: Discovering Yoga

Part IV: Discovering Karma and Past Lives

Part V: Discovering ESP

Part VI: Discovering Enlightenment

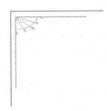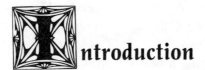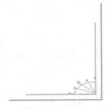

Introduction

I t was the height of the spiritual revolution in Berkeley, California: 1967. Flower children and hippies abounded. At age nineteen I was one of them.

What changed my life was the day I entered a meditation center. A faint fragrance of flowers, incense, and camphor lingered in the air. The photograph on the wall was somehow familiar, yet I'd never met the longhaired, bearded *guru* ("one who brings light to the darkness" in Sanskrit) dressed in white silk robes with coral beads around his neck. I immediately fell in (spiritual) love.

For the next twenty-one years I studied and resided with this guru in his *ashrams* (spiritual communities) in India, Switzerland, Spain, Austria, Italy, in the Himalayas, the Alps, and secluded areas of the United States. For seven of those years I was on his personal staff. His name was Maharishi Mahesh Yogi, founder of Transcendental Meditation, the largest meditation organization in the world.

My daily experience during those years consisted of deep meditation and Yoga. I meditated up to twenty hours a day, sometimes entering my room and not appearing until eight weeks later. I went into silence and didn't utter a word for up to four months at a time. I was an introvert—and that's definitely an understatement.

Every day meditation brought me to the state of *samadhi* (equipoise) and *satchitananda* (absolute bliss consciousness), the goals of yoga. This was a more profound experience of inner peace and deep silence than I could have ever imagined.

After spending twenty years with my eyes closed, however, I woke up one day to realize I wasn't a spiritual person. How could I regularly attain the goal of Yoga, the sublime state of samadhi, and not be spiritual? Somehow, I did.

You might define a spiritual person as kind, generous, charitable, gentle, compassionate, loving, and patient. I wasn't any of these. In fact, I was a "b" with an "itch." I looked around the ashram and found an abundance of meditators who were also selfish, narcissistic, impatient, rude, arrogant, pretentious, caustic, and immensely fearful, even to the point of paranoia.

Something was missing. Although I experienced deep meditation and fulfillment in the state of samadhi, that wasn't enough. The impersonal deep silence of satchitananda didn't make me more loving, although it brought inner peace. I wasn't aware I could experience a richer, fuller experience of my divine nature—the personal aspect of Spirit.

Happily, luckily, through meeting Dr. Peter Meyer and becoming involved with his organization, Teaching of Intuitional Metaphysics, I learned how to contact and communicate with the indwelling, loving, divine presence, the intimate, personal aspect of the divine. This was an amazing transformation that opened my mind and heart to a myriad of joyous adventures into inner space that I want to share with you.

Therefore, I've written this book to help you explore both the impersonal absolute, the sublime goal of Yoga, called satchitananda, and also the personal aspects of your divine higher self. The teaching that I founded, Divine Revelation, helps anyone listen to the "still small voice" of divine intuition within and to use it in a practical way to solve everyday problems, receive divine guidance, love, healing, and inspiration, and be led by Spirit in daily life.

In this book you'll learn how to safely and easily contact both the impersonal and personal aspects of Spirit, to practice deep meditation, to perfect methods of Yoga, develop intuition, and fulfill desires. It also makes East Indian philosophy and mysticism accessible to everyone. This book is for both beginners as well as those who are more advanced on their spiritual paths. It will help you realize who you truly are and attain spiritual enlightenment, the goal of human life.

This book is divided into six parts. Part I is about realizing the glory of your higher self. Part II helps you meditate and provides a simple guided meditation you can start right away. Part III provides many Yogic practices to culture both body and breath. Part IV is about fulfilling desires and manifesting your dreams. Part V helps you develop your intuition. Part VI brings wisdom of spiritual enlightenment and Eastern philosophy.

Each chapter begins with a "chapter affirmation," that you can repeat aloud several times during the day. This will help you realize your true nature as you read the book and use its techniques.

To my mind, meditation is not only a way to awaken your spirituality and conscious awareness, but also improve the quality of life on the planet. Harmony of mind and body, brought about by deep meditation, creates an atmosphere of love and peace that can generate planetary transformation much more effectively than any treaty or ambassador of good will.

By listening to your inner voice and following its guidance, you'll be led to your highest purpose and destiny, which is of highest good, not only for yourself, but also for everyone and everything. If enough people were to meditate, this world would transform from suffering and chaos to the most glorious age of enlightenment in recorded history. This book will show you how.

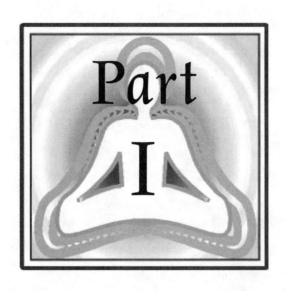

Part I

Discovering Your
Higher Self

Chapter 1

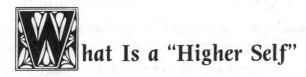

hat Is a "Higher Self"
Anyway?

In This Chapter:
- Asking Questions about Spiritual Development.
- Taking the "Meditation IQ Test."
- Getting Acquainted with Your Higher Self.

Chapter Affirmation:
"I AM a radiant being of pure light."

A homemaker from Staten Island, New York came to me to learn how to meditate. Like so many of us, she was seeking an unmistakable, concrete signal to help her identify whether she was in contact with her higher self. When I led her into meditation and asked her to describe her experience, she said, "Peace." I asked her to take a few deep breaths and then repeated my question. She still answered, "Peace." This went on a few more times. Finally I asked her where this "peace" was located. She promptly replied, "It's that feeling of having a cloak around my shoulders that everyone gets when they meditate." I explained that this feeling of a cloak was her own unique experience, different from what others experience when they meditate.

This story illustrates a simple point—we all have preconceptions and misconceptions about meditation. There's always room for learning, even for experienced meditators. You might be surprised at what this book has to offer.

Others of you may be curious, yet completely unfamiliar with the territory of meditation and spiritual development. Therefore we'll begin with the basics and answer a few of your questions.

FAQ's About Spiritual Development

Q: I don't understand the concepts of meditation, enlightenment, psychic phenomena, or supernatural experiences. Can I learn about these?

A: This book provides knowledge of the basics as well as surprising information that experts in this field are unaware of. Therefore, you can gain even greater understanding than many street-wise metaphysicians.

Q: I tried meditation, but it didn't work for me. Can I learn to do it?

A: This book will help you meditate easily and effortlessly with sure-fire techniques that work even for beginners.

Q: I have no confidence in my intuition. What can I do about this?

A: Here you can learn simple, step-by-step methods to help you develop and use your intuition and ESP power.

Q: When I have inner experiences, I pretend they didn't happen.

A: With this book you can begin to understand, accept, and have confidence in your spiritual experiences.

Q: I feel overwhelmed by the maze of occult offerings in pop culture today.

A: In this book you can learn to distinguish between spiritual and mental experiences and avoid the pitfalls of psychic delusion.

Q: I feel overly sensitive to people and things around me.

A: This book offers powerful techniques to heal negative influences and prevent harm from future influences.

Q: I don't want to work at hard-to-follow disciplines.

A: This book is easy to understand, with simple-to-learn methods that require no previous experience, background, training, or knowledge.

Q: **I don't like rules, regulations, cults, and organizations.**

A: These methods impose no restrictions and are compatible with other forms of meditation and religious philosophies, lifestyles, and personal beliefs.

Q: **I want to grow spiritually, yet I have no idea how to begin.**

A: This book can inspire you to a more spiritually directed life, beginning with the basics. How far you progress on your spiritual path is entirely up to you.

Test Your Meditation IQ

Perhaps you feel that since you have studied meditation and spiritual development for decades, this book is too elementary. Even if you're an expert, this test just might stump you:

1. **What is your higher self?**
   A. The divine within me.
   B. My soul.
   C. The good part of myself.
   D. Myself after death.
   E. Part of myself that's above my body.
   F. A '60s flashback.

2. **What is meditation?**
   A. Concentration of mind.
   B. Contemplating a profound statement.
   C. Quieting mind and body.
   D. Going into a trance.
   E. Repeating a mantra.
   F. Something naughty you do with the door closed.

3. **What is a mantra?**
   A. Any word used in meditation.
   B. A meaningless sound that's chanted.
   C. A name or phrase used as an invocation.

D. Japa.

E. A prayer.

F. A secret handshake.

4. **What is samadhi?**

A. Stillness and equanimity of mind and body.

B. A yoga exercise.

C. An East Indian philosophy.

D. Freedom from karma.

E. Meditation.

F. Saturday in the south of France.

5. **What is yoga?**

A. A specific type of exercise program.

B. To yoke.

C. Getting into certain postures.

D. Eastern philosophy.

E. Breathing exercises.

F. Booboo's pal.

6. **What is kundalini?**

A. Enlightenment.

B. Mystic energy coil.

C. A sign that I'm experiencing higher consciousness.

D. Sexual orgasm.

E. An Indian goddess.

F. A pasta.

7. **What is a chakra?**

A. A wheel.

B. The center of the body.

C. A clairvoyant sight.

D. When it opens, I become enlightened.

E. A nerve ending.

F. That awful screeching blackboard sound.

8. What is karma?

    A. Getting back what I deserve.

    B. Action.

    C. Reward or punishment for past lives.

    D. Good or bad luck.

    E. Reincarnation.

    F. My mother's Ford Taurus.

9. What is dharma?

    A. What I should be doing.

    B. The path for more highly evolved people.

    C. Ethical morality.

    D. My career.

    E. Following my true heart's desires.

    F. An expletive.

10. What is unconscious trance mediumship?

    A. Letting divine beings take over your body.

    B. Letting unkown entities take over your body.

    C. Demonic possession.

    D. Spiritualism.

    E. Getting higher knowledge from entities.

    F. Sleeping through your trans-Atlantic ocean voyage.

11. What is an astral entity?

    A. A demon.

    B. A person who died.

    C. An evil spirit.

    D. An earthbound spirit.

    E. A higher being who gives information through channeling.

    F. A baseball player for the Houston team.

12. What is intuition?

    A. Insight.

    B. Something women have.

C. Psychic powers.

D. Predicting the future.

E. Telepathy.

F. A hospital, school, or prison.

13. What is ESP?

A. Seeing, hearing, and feeling things without the senses.

B. Getting higher knowledge.

C. Moving things telekinetically.

D. Predicting the future.

E. Having subtle sensory experiences inwardly.

F. A cable TV network.

14. Who is called a psychic?

A. A person who may or may not have ESP.

B. A person who knows the future.

C. A person with supernormal powers.

D. A person who reads cards.

E. An astrologer.

F. Someone who makes money on TV.

15. What is a guru?

A. A cult leader.

B. One who brings light to the darkness.

C. A person who should be worshipped.

D. A teacher to whom I should surrender.

E. A teacher who knows better than me what is best for me.

F. The past tense of goyim.

16. What is maya?

A. Being ensnared by a beautiful woman.

B. Being worldly.

C. Being materialistic.

D. Not knowing about enlightenment.

E. That which doesn't exist.

F. Famous African-American poetess.

17. What is reincarnation?

A. Transmigration of the soul.

B. Being born again as a lower life form.

C. My past lives.

D. Predestination.

E. Punishment for bad karma.

F. Giving me a flower that someone gave to you.

18. What is enlightenment?

A. Knowing who I really am.

B. Being a guru.

C. Being higher than other people.

D. Freedom from all responsibilities.

E. Release from the world.

F. Finally losing that ten pounds.

The answers to this quiz are 1:A, 2:C, 3:C, 4:A, 5:B, 6:B, 7:A, 8:B, 9:E, 10:B, 11:D, 12:A, 13:E, 14:A, 15:B, 16:E, 17:A, and 18:A.

- If you got 18 right, your spiritual IQ is 200. You don't need to read this book. You should write your own.

- If you got 14-17 right, you're a DOCTOR OF SPIRITUALITY. You have tremendous insight into spiritual development and your spiritual IQ is 175.

- If you got 10-13 right, you're a MASTER OF SPIRITUALITY. You know a lot, but you have a few things to learn. Your spiritual IQ is 150.

- If you got 5-9 right, you're a BACHELOR OF SPIRITUALITY. You still know a lot, but you have more to learn. Your spiritual IQ is 125.

- If you got 1-4 right, congratulations, the odds are with you. You've successfully proven that random selection works. Your spiritual IQ is 100.

Are you surprised at some of the answers on the quiz? That's because so many myths surround these words. Having some familiarity with esoteric terms is not the same as understanding them deeply. As you read

Exploring Meditation, you'll acquire profound insight into these terms. Let's begin by answering the first "Meditation IQ Test" question, namely, "What is your higher self?"

FAQ's about Your Higher Self

Q: **What is a "higher self," and does it have meaning for me in my busy life?**

A: Jerome Ballantine, A New York fashion executive, told me recently:

> "In meditation, in my inner eye I saw my higher self as a tall, radiant being in yellow robes with penetrating large brown eyes. Identifying himself as Sananda, he led me through a doorway into a vast space. With stars and galaxies all around me, I ascended into a realm of light and left time and space behind. I became infinitely expanded, and the universe became a tiny dot within me. I was filled with great happiness and peace. For a time I became one with the universe and completely forgot my body and everything else. As a result of this experience, my higher self is with me daily, granting me constant support, comfort, guidance, love, and protection."

Even busy executives can have profound experiences of their higher self. Not just isolated flash-in-the-pan phenomena, these are profound, meaningful occurrences that affect every aspect of daily life.

The higher self is a part of you that usually remains hidden from view. It's thought of as your spiritual self or the higher aspect of your being. Yet most people misunderstand it and don't realize its significance.

Q: **In what way does an experience of my higher self have meaning to me?**

A: Experiencing your higher self can literally transform the way you see yourself, how you relate to your environment, and how you interact with others. It can augment your career success and dramatically improve your level of self-confidence and measure of happiness.

Q: **Why and how can my higher self transform my life?**

A: Getting in touch with your higher self awakens hidden aspects of yourself that haven't yet been brought to conscious awareness. These higher aspects, with special properties and abilities, can exercise your mind in new ways. Like an out-of-use muscle that has atrophied, your higher self needs to be used. Then it becomes an ally that transforms your life into something new. You become more happy, successful, radiant, beautiful, and fulfilled.

Q: How can I contact my higher self?

A: Through meditation you can connect with your higher self. By quieting your mind, you can recognize who the higher self is and what it can do for you. In this book you'll learn some practical ways to do this.

Q: How does my higher self work?

A: Your higher self works with your ego-self to carry out the process of your spiritual awakening in consciousness. You're constantly reinventing yourself into higher states of awareness every moment, opening to understandings you weren't previously aware of. Each new day brings a higher state of consciousness than the day before. You're waking up day by day, as you recognize the perfection and truth of your being.

Q: What is the purpose of my life?

A: Your life purpose is to enjoy greater happiness and express more of who you really are. Who you really are and who you think you are may be very different from each other. For you are an enlightened, spiritually awake, highly tuned, powerful being, at one with the universe and with your divine self.

Q: How can I begin to realize who I really am?

A: Your higher self will teach you who you really are once you experience it directly in meditation and communicate with it. But this must be a direct experience, not an intellectualization. Only by going direct to the source, without any intermediary, can you realize your true self.

Q: What benefits can I receive through contacting my higher self?

A: ▪ Love.
Contact with your higher self brings more love into your life, since you drop personality façades that previously created walls between yourself and others.

- Power.
  You also become more powerful and effective, since you're tapping an unlimited gold mind of power and wisdom at the center of your being.

- Happiness.
  Since the experience of the higher self is great joy and deep satisfaction, you naturally become happier and more fulfilled.

- Energy.
  You have more energy, since you stop trying so hard to please others and relax into being more natural and true to yourself.

- Wisdom.
  You develop your full mental potential when you awaken to the innate wisdom and inner knowing of your higher self.

- Less Stress.
  You reduce stress and tension and increase well-being and contentment, since you become more self-contained and self-reliant.

- Health.
  Your health improves because as you start to identify with your higher self, you become more physically relaxed and psychologically balanced.

- Contentment.
  You feel more content when you attune to the higher self because you gain trust in the universe to provide for your needs.

- Peace of Mind.
  You experience greater peace of mind, since you find what you've been seeking all your life, even if you didn't know it at the time.

Q: What is the nature of my higher self?

A: Your higher self is your true nature—the divine within. It may be completely unlike what you believe yourself to be. In fact, you may not recognize it as your self when you first encounter it. You might even think it's someone or something other than you. But in reality it's the true nature of your being—beautiful, free, loving, generous, joyous, wise, and creative—the divine in action, expressing itself as yourself.

Q: What does my higher self look like, and how does it feel?

A: Your higher self is a radiant, beautiful light-being. It has no heavy mass like your earthly physical body. It may be a myriad of beautiful colors and isn't confined to the space or even the time where your physical body is located. Deep in meditation you'll experience your higher self as a sense of happiness, fulfillment, wholeness, and profound peace.

It's multi-leveled and multi-faceted. Your higher self is not your human personality and not just your soul. It includes layer upon layer of dimensions. All aspects of the divine abide within you. At the heart of your very nature dwells the higher power (in whatever form you believe that to be), in all its multifarious forms.

You'll experience your higher self in a way that's suited to you and makes you comfortable. For example, if you happen to be Jewish, you may not want to meet Jesus during your trips to inner space. If you're Catholic, you may feel uncomfortable meeting Buddha. (But don't be too surprised if you happen to run across them at some point down the road.)

Beyond all your multidimensional aspects there's an even deeper aspect—the absolute—beyond all forms and phenomena of the material world and even beyond the celestial realm. But now we're getting ahead of ourselves. We'll explore more about this later on.

Q: Why do I need to know this stuff?

A: If you don't learn it now, it's okay. It doesn't matter. Eventually you'll come back to it in the future, either in this life or another life (whoops, yep, reincarnation). Somewhere along your path you'll have to stop the madness of living in the illusion of *maya* (identifying yourself as your ego) and wake up to who you really are. It's just that simple.

> *"The question 'Who am I?' is the one that annihilates all others."*
> —Ramana Maharishi

Chapter 2

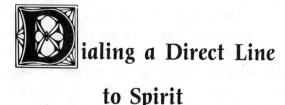

ialing a Direct Line
to Spirit

In This Chapter:
- Defining "Spirit" and "God."
- Learning to Communicate with Spirit.
- Contacting the Divine through Meditation.

Chapter Affirmation:
"I AM perfection everywhere now."

Y ou may be wondering, "Why should I learn to meditate? What's in it for me?" The answer is simple: There's a lot more than you could ever imagine.

Your higher self wants to know you intimately and communicate with you daily. But you may not be aware it's available to you. Perhaps you think only prophets touched with a divine magic wand can contact their higher selves. Yet you're just as capable of doing this as any great saint. Are you surprised? If so, you have company—most people believe only the "elect" are worthy to communicate with Spirit.

By practicing meditation as outlined in this book, you can contact your higher self and communicate with Spirit. While we're at it, let's define what we mean by "Spirit" or "God." (By the way, they're the same.)

What Is Spirit?

"Spirit" is an aspect of you that is divine—not limited by any religion, lifestyle, personal belief, or denomination. It's your sense of wonder when you see a beautiful rose and smell its fragrance, when you feel the warm wind caressing your face and blowing your hair, when you watch the relentless ebb and flow of the ocean's waves crashing on the shore.

Who doesn't appreciate this awesome creation—from the magnificent starry skies to the silence of damp, mossy leaf-laden trees in a dense forest floor? Every time you see your baby smile or the light in your lover's eyes, there Spirit is. Spirit is all around you, in every song, every word, and every thought. You don't have to go far to find Spirit. It's right here, right now.

"God" or "Spirit" is defined as your higher power, in whatever form you personally believe that to be. Right now you might not know "who" or "what" God is. You may not even believe God exists. After all, He/She/It hasn't been measured scientifically. And today we're all devout worshippers of science, aren't we? At least it seems so.

If I had to quantify Spirit scientifically, the mathematical concept "infinity" would suffice. This concept, although incomprehensible to the linear left-brain, appeals to the higher mind. All you mathematicians may object to being branded metaphysicians, but, well, that's just the way it is. You might also think of Spirit as that elusive "unified field" that all physicists since Einstein have struggled to locate.

In any case, you don't have to believe in God to get benefits from meditation. During meditation, *belief* is inconsequential. You're *directly experiencing* Spirit, rather than thinking about it.

That's what you're going to learn from this book: how to experience Spirit directly. Then you'll know what Spirit is from the inside and won't need it defined. Your sense of wonder will be a direct experience.

Where Is Spirit Located?

You may not be aware of it, but your spiritual self is guiding your destiny right now. You're in continual contact with Spirit. It's the very blood that rushes through your arteries, the life force flowing in and out with each breath. Without Spirit, you wouldn't be alive.

Probably you've heard "God is within," even from the Bible: "The kingdom of God is within you."[1] Perhaps you don't believe it. If you don't, consider this: Do you believe divine Spirit is everywhere? If you answered yes, then, by deduction, you'll agree that Spirit is in all things, even you. Could Spirit be everywhere except inside you? Are you exempt?

Fess up; you're somewhere, right? If you're somewhere, then Spirit is also there. Guess you'll have to admit that one!

Now that you realize divine Spirit is within, I suppose you'll agree that Spirit is approachable rather than inaccessible. It's only logical that if Spirit is inside, then He/She/It must be easy to talk to, or at least capable of communicating with to some degree.

How Can I Communicate With Spirit?

You've probably talked to Spirit all your life. It started when you were young. These are probably one-way conversations. You talk, and Spirit listens. (At least you hope so.) But did Spirit speak back? If so, and if you told anyone, then you might be reading this book in Bellevue Hospital, because you'd be diagnosed as psychotic. Talking to God? What?

Well, it's true. Anyone who admits to either seeing or hearing God is considered either saintly or insane, depending on whether that person is a monk or a homeless person. Society thinks if you talk to God, it's called "prayer," but if God talks to you, it's called "schizophrenia."

Think about it. As a child, did you learn to experience God directly? Were you taught to hear the divine voice within your heart?

If you were raised in a "normal" family, you learned that God might or might not hear your prayers, and you may or may not get them answered. God might reward or punish you, depending on His mood. Why wouldn't you think all conversations with God are one-way conversations? You pray and that's it. Finished. No way could Spirit ever talk back.

Then after you die maybe, just maybe, you will get to meet God. Perhaps, if you're really lucky, you could have a "near-death" or "out-of-body" experience while still alive. Then you could experience Spirit directly. Otherwise, you're out of luck.

This book flies in the face of all such beliefs that Spirit is far away and elusive. Instead, it maintains you can see, hear, feel, and directly experience the divine, right here, right now. You don't need to die to do this. There's no one who can't do this.

I'm not claiming that you'll communicate directly with Spirit from just reading this book. But if you follow the techniques outlined here, and if you practice meditation regularly, you can have genuine divine experiences. You might also achieve direct, two-way conversations with God. You'll learn how later in this book.

Is Spirit Attainable?

Imagine I show you a strawberry and say, "Look at this beautiful berry. See the rich red color and these yellowish seeds. See the silky green stem and leaves. How delicious, so sweet and scrumptious." If you never tasted a strawberry, you wouldn't know what I was talking about. That is, until you took a bite and ate it. Then you'd know for sure what a strawberry is.

Similarly, many spiritual teachers tell their students how wonderful Spirit is. But those same teachers can't give their students direct experience of this loving, divine presence. How can those who've never tasted the strawberry themselves possibly help others taste it?

Intellectualizing the reality of the divine presence isn't enough. Describing Spirit is insufficient. It must become a reality of everyday life. How can you taste the strawberry and communicate with Spirit directly?

Can only special "holy" people (who lived at least two thousand years ago in some faraway land) communicate with Spirit? Ancient prophets are placed high on a pedestal, even deified. These lofty saints, sages, seers, and holy men (emphasis on the word "men") somehow managed to get their foot into the divine door. Their revelations are supposedly the only direct "Word of God"—the Holy Scriptures.

What about the rest of us? Have saintly people signed an exclusive contract with God? Or can ordinary people experience Spirit? Are we banished from the holy kingdom? That's what many religious institutions would have us believe.

Contrary to popular belief, God isn't a capricious being, limited by time or space. Spirit is present everywhere and can be in many places and times at once. Divinity places no conditions or regulations, doesn't play favorites, and has no bias toward one race or religion.

Even though religious scriptures state that Spirit is immanent, in fact, the very source of our being, still we're unconvinced. Why? Because religious institutions today don't seem to believe their original scriptures. We've been conditioned to think that pastors and churches have the only direct line to Spirit.

Such a myth is perpetuated for one reason only—control. After all, what is the incentive for religious organizations to help us have direct divine communication? None. It's not in their interest. If they were successful in this endeavor, soon they would be out of business. If a retailer gave his customers a way to buy products wholesale, where would he be?

Well, just think of this book as a wholesaler in the divine-revelation business. You can go direct and cut out the middleman. Don't get me wrong. I'm not trying to malign religious institutions. I'm just helping you see your own beauty and power. You're a radiant being with unlimited strength, definitely capable and worthy to experience Spirit directly.

Yes, it's possible to experience divine Spirit anytime, 24 hours a day—through meditation. Happily, many ancient teachings of the East have been exported to the West. You're the recipient of this bounty. You can fill the bucket from the well and drink your fill. Since the 1960s, many enlightened spiritual masters have freely bestowed secret knowledge on just about anyone who wants it. I've had the fortunate opportunity to study with some of them. Whatever I've learned, I willingly give to anyone who has a sincere desire to use the knowledge.

Here is what the great masters of all ages say: You're not the small, insignificant being you thought you were. You have a destiny and purpose beyond your seemingly insecure ego. You have a divine center that's vast, profound, and infinite. Your higher self is the source of power, energy, and love, and is definitely worth contacting.

Your higher self is eager to give you everything. It can help you in daily life; it can heal you and fulfill your true desires. Only you must open to it. Spirit is continually knocking on the door, waiting for you to open to its magnificent radiance. Once you open it, your life is transformed. You experience greater happiness and fulfillment. By letting go of old habits that bound you to the past, a brighter future opens.

Meditation is definitely the key to this opening. Without meditation, it's difficult for the average person to get anywhere with spiritual development. That's because inner quietude is a prerequisite for experiencing the divine. This tranquil state can't be achieved by obsessively following worldly pursuits.

It's necessary to pause, take a moment out of your day, get quiet, and reflect. Meditation is the way to do this. It quiets the mind and body so you can contact your higher self and experience divine wisdom, perfect love, and inner knowing.

What Is Meditation?

Deep meditation is a technique of quieting the mind and body. Your mind settles to tranquillity, and your body becomes still. Your body is relaxed, often more deeply than sleep, yet your mind is more alert than wakefulness. Your awareness expands. Losing awareness of body and surroundings, you get absorbed in the experience of infinite bliss.

The reason you forget your surroundings is that your higher self strongly holds your attention during meditation. This is called "concentration." Yet it's not concentration in the sense you probably think. Concentration is usually associated with taking a test or memorizing something. What I mean is during meditation your mind becomes focused on the self.

Just as, while watching an absorbing movie, you're so engrossed that you forget everything else; similarly, in meditation you're so enthralled that you forget everything else. Your higher self is the most fascinating object of attention that could possibly engage your mind. That's concentration.

Nothing is more interesting than direct contact with Spirit. Let's say you've always worn costume jewelry and never saw real jewelry. Then someone gives you the Crown Jewels to wear. These precious gemstones and real gold are so radiant and filled with beauty that you're completely enamored with them. Now you'll never go back to imitation paste jewelry. Similarly, when you experience the real thing within your soul, your mind is completely absorbed. Once you have that undeniable experience, you'll never forget it.

Deep meditation is a way to expand your mind. It provides a wide-angle lens for you to view your life. Rather than getting wrapped up in trivial details, you open to a higher perspective. Worries simply melt away, and after you come out of meditation, you feel refreshed, reinvigorated, and ready to go. No longer bound by anxieties, you move forward with confidence.

It's as if during meditation you leave the past behind, and when you come out, you're reborn. In this way you could liken meditation to sleep. You go to bed tired and then wake up refreshed. Yet meditation is more profound than sleep. Not only does it bring release of daily stresses; it also heals deep patterns and traumas. More importantly, it takes your mind to higher awareness and direct contact with Spirit.

"Who" or "What" Do You Contact during Meditation?

The technique of meditation taught in this book is a safe process. It's a way to establish a direct link with Spirit, like talking on the phone. You may experience this communication in many different ways. For example, you may:

- See inspiring inner spiritual visions, such as images of Jesus or Moses, with your inner eye.

- Hear messages from the divine voice within and receive words of comfort, love, and inspiration with your inner ear.

- Taste or smell divine fragrances or flavors that uplift your conscious awareness, such as sweet flowers or fruits.

- Feel experiences of touching the divine nature and receive awakening of divine energy within your body.

- Go beyond all sensory experience to the sublime realm of pure bliss consciousness.

When you have these experiences, your link to the divine may be strong, like a satellite hook-up, or weak and narrow, like an extension cord in your home. Meditating regularly widens and deepens that connection, like a direct cable to the Internet. Don't worry if at first your experiences leave something to be desired. With time and patience you'll have the divine experiences you seek, even greater than you can imagine—simply by asking.

Who do you contact in meditation? Hopefully, if you don't have your wires crossed, you'll be in touch with your higher self and aspects of Spirit within. These are attributes of the divine personified in various forms. Aspects of divinity, such as Holy Spirit, Jesus, Mary, Allah, Quan Yin, Jehovah, Krishna, Shiva, Lakshmi, Buddha, and so forth, are all available in "inner space." And you'll meet them.

You can also contact your higher self, or *Atman,* the "I AM" self—the aspect of self that Moses contacted when he saw the burning bush. This divine voice said to Moses, "I AM that I AM."[2]

You might also experience an aspect of yourself called *Brahman,* above all personifications. Beyond relative forms and phenomena of the universe, Brahman is truly the mathematician's concept of infinity. It is the impersonal aspect of the divine, without name or form.

What's It Like to Contact Spirit?

Your experience of Spirit will be entirely unique. However, there are some common denominators that most meditators experience. You'll probably feel deep inner peace, relaxation, happiness, contentment and fulfillment. You'll be in balance, unity, and wholeness.

When contacting aspects of the divine, a great surge of spiritual awakening and divine grace may overcome you. You might feel touched by Spirit. Maybe you'll feel loved, protected and cared for—safe in divine arms and secure in the experience that you're "home again."

No separation will exist between you and Spirit. You'll see yourself as part of the divine rather than an isolated entity. In tune with the divine, your mind will be connected to Spirit. Your thoughts will be divine thoughts rather than thoughts of your limited ego, and you'll begin to identify with your higher self.

What does this mean? If you were asked the question, "Who are you?" you might answer: "I am so-and-so years old, such-and-such height and weight, with these hair and eyes, born this date, with this job, these hobbies, and so-much money in the bank. I live in this house, drive this car, have this job, this wife, these children, this education. I follow this religion, belong to this political party and am spiritual—or not—and busy myself with these hobbies. That's who I am."

But is that who you really are? Are you solely identified by your history and material things?

Once you contact your higher self, you identify yourself differently. No longer does your identity depend on outer trappings of body and material life. Now you identify with something else—your higher self. You're not just this mind, this body, this bank account. You now awaken to the realization of who you are—a divine child of the living God, Spirit in physical form.

"You Are God"

"What? I am God? Nonsense. Isn't God that big man in the sky with the white beard? He's the creator of the universe. I didn't create anything. I'm a lowly, insignificant, powerless creature. God is all-powerful and omniscient. It's blasphemy to say that I am God."

This may be what you're thinking. You might see yourself as insignificant. But that's not how God sees it. You were made in God's image and likeness.[3] You were given a great gift—free will. This gift has made you into the semblance of God. However, you must use this god-like gift well, to realize you're like the almighty, rather than insignificant and powerless.

God doesn't make anyone powerless. By using your own god-like free will, you choose to make yourself powerless. In fact, you have total freedom to be whatever you want. You can be powerful, powerless, or anything in between. Along with God, you co-created your own universe. That's why you're god-like.

Stand up and end all the self-deprecating nonsense. You aren't a small creature. Within you is unlimited power, energy, and intelligence which you can tap and utilize daily. You already have everything you need and all you could ever desire. You can complain about your problems, but the biggest problem is that you created your problems yourself. There's no one else to blame. Neither is there any point in blaming yourself. Just realize that you created your own world and therefore have the power to change it.

In this book you'll be given tools to help you significantly transform your life for the better. You can make use of these techniques and stop bewailing the unhappy fate of your present circumstances.

"There is no reason to suffer. Life is meant to enjoy. Life is bliss." That's what my guru used to say. By practicing meditation and transforming your life, you can make this aphorism a reality. I realize it sounds Pollyanna, but, in fact, I believe meditation is the cure for all suffering. After practicing meditation since 1967, I can confidently assert it's a panacea for all problems—emotional, mental, physical, material, and spiritual.

"Let me know myself, Lord, and I shall know Thee."
—St.Augustine

Chapter 3

 User-friendly Guide to Your Self

In This Chapter:
- Discovering Who You Really Are.
- Letting Go of Illusions.
- A Road Map to Your Inner Life.

Chapter Affirmation:
"I AM the light that God is."
—John 14:12

Who am I? This is the age-old question spiritual seekers have asked centuries. The ancient prophets and scriptures provide an answer that might surprise you. You are, in fact, created in the very image and likeness of God. That means you are loving, powerful, and almighty, as the Creator is, and you can manifest miracles. Jesus once said: "Greater works than these shall [ye] do."[1]

You may not feel capable of working miracles. You might consider yourself insignificant and powerless. Yet that inconsequential person is not who you really are. Within you is a powerful connection to divine Spirit. When you become aware of that contact and use it consciously, you can do miracles, even "greater works than these."

Many of you consider yourself "average," with no special qualities to distinguish yourself. When you compare yourself to more talented, more popular, happy, wealthy, healthy, or beautiful people, perhaps your limitations glare at you like a bare light bulb dangling from a cracked ceiling.

It's easy to imagine how puny and trivial we are, in contrast to great artists, authors, playwrights, musicians, scientists, athletes, healers, business people, inventors, geniuses, and other luminaries. Yet the inner genius—the true you—can be cultivated and expressed. Just let go of the illusion about who you think you are.

"Who you think you are" consists of your ego-identity and limited beliefs. "Who you really are" is more magnificent than you could ever imagine. You're a powerful, divine, wondrous being of wisdom and love, an unlimited, radiant being of pure light.

Where do our limited beliefs originate? Why do we consider ourselves inferior? The answer lies in our past.

What's Your Self-Image?

While your mother was suckling you or father was bouncing you on his knee, they were writing the script of your life. Most likely your parents taught you the same things their parents taught them, which their parents taught them, and so forth, as long as the world has existed. A group of fundamental human beliefs has been handed down, generation to generation. What are these beliefs? Are they true? Here are a few of them:

1. God is far away, impossible to attain.
2. God has no time for us.
3. Life is a struggle.
4. Humans must suffer.
5. Sinful people go to hell.
6. Money is the root of all evil.
7. There isn't enough to go around.
8. Spiritual people must be poor.
9. The rich can't be spiritual.
10. The poor are virtuous.

11. The rich take advantage of the poor.
12. It's sinful to earn money as a healer or spiritual teacher.
13. People with ESP are in league with the devil.
14. Women don't deserve what men have.
15. Women must be submissive.
16. Women are only valuable when they're young.
17. The elderly are useless.
18. Men must be aggressive.
19. Men must take charge.
20. Men must fight.
21. It's okay for men to be sexually promiscuous, but not okay for women.
22. Better safe than sorry.
23. Don't take risks.
24. Don't deviate.
25. Be like everyone else.

Many of us don't question these fundamental beliefs. We go about our lives, half-asleep, and don't question anything. But is it possible that some of these beliefs aren't true? Do we have more power than we thought?

Look at yourself in the mirror. That's right. Go over to the mirror right now and look at yourself. Do you like what you see, or are you ashamed? Are you happy and proud to be you, or do you look away after a glance?

Your self-image comes from a variety of sources. Your parents were your first teachers. Whatever blatant or subtle messages they imparted defined your self-image. If your mother constantly said, "You're fat," then wouldn't losing weight be difficult? If your father blithely declared, "You'll never amount to anything," then wouldn't success elude you? If your grandmother harped on your mistakes, then wouldn't you either feel like an oaf—or perhaps become one?

Your beliefs, as taught by your relatives, determine not only your self-image, but also your destiny. Similarly, your teachers, religion, peers, society, and the media—all these factors contribute to your self-concept.

If you're continually barraged with television images of thin, blond, Barbie-doll-like women and tall, buff, muscle-bound men, what happens when you gaze into the mirror at a short, fat brunette who doesn't fit the standard? Do you see the beauty within? Or do you buy the idea that's been shoved down your throat by the media?

The bad news is that you may have bought the messages from your environment. Perhaps you clutch onto these ideas with vigor. The good news is you don't have to. Why? Because of a wonderful gift from the Creator—free will. You can either hold onto those old ideas, or you can replace them with new ones.

Now let's go back to the mirror. That's right. Go back and look again. But this time, say to that mirror, out loud, "I love you." In fact, it would be an excellent idea to say that affirmation to your mirror every day. And mean it. More about affirmations later in the book.

Am I Less than Others?

You're a multi-faceted, multi-dimensional, magnificent being of love, light, strength, and energy. You're as good as any other person on this planet, and everyone else is as good as you. No one is superior or inferior. Humans maintain a sort of caste system with some people on top of the ladder and others at the bottom. But that system is an illusion.

Differences in philosophy, political views, and religion perpetuate class and rank. People often struggle to prove they're right and kill anyone who disagrees. Philosophical or political groups believe with fervor in the merit of their world-view. Fanaticism finds ingenious ways to prevent others from expressing an opinion. Distinctions in race or religion prove ample fodder for abuse and war—even wholesale slaughter. Ethnic cleansing and terrorism are the outcome of such abuse, taken to the nth degree.

The ruling class places itself above others, abuses power, and grants itself the divine right of superiority. The lower class prides itself as the underdog, blames its problems on the wealthy, and relishes its self-righteous victim-hood.

In such an atmosphere of class differences and philosophical disagreements, it's nearly impossible to avoid beliefs of superiority and inferiority, even at an early age. As teenagers, we learn all too painfully, as we vie for popularity with jocks and cheerleaders, or struggle with being a nerd. We also learn early about the advantages of physical beauty and disadvantages of ugliness.

But are we so different from each other? Or does something underlie our humanness that makes us similar? Is there unity amongst the diversity of race, class, religion, and political opinion?

The divine presence, the spiritual center of our being, unifies all diversity. We all belong to that all-embracing presence. As we experience that directly, we discover what binds us together and let go of differences.

Hope for the planet lies in individuals realizing the fundamental truth that we are all one. We're not so much separate individuals, classes, races, and religions, as we are the same wholeness that underlies and pervades everything.

Once you experience this, through meditation, you can envision the possibility of world peace, harmony, and happiness. How? By many individuals waking up to who they really are.

Beyond Duality

Let's delve into the question "Who am I?" by starting with the oneness underlying and pervading the universe. That oneness is the "absolute," beyond duality of relative life. What do you see around you? A world of differences, beginning with the most fundamental: light/dark, male/female, hot/cold, black/white, bright/dull, sad/happy, love/hate, yin/yang. This is "duality." The world of dualism is the "relative" field.

But there are two aspects of life: relative and absolute. The ultimate reality of oneness is beyond the "pairs of opposites" of relativity. The absolute is said to be "one without a second" and is called *Brahman* in Sanskrit.

What is the absolute? Can it be experienced directly? "Perfection everywhere now" is one way to describe it. You might think that perfection is impossible and doesn't exist. And you'd be right. It doesn't exist in the relative field, where we live. But it does exist in oneness at the center of your being.

Beyond your body, mind, emotions and all duality, at the core of your being is an absolute field of pure consciousness, pure intelligence, pure beingness without judgment, fear, hate, or even love, joy, or happiness. The absolute lies beyond all relative experiences, such as love and hate, which can only be defined by their opposites.

Beyond all relative experiences is that which needs nothing to define it: the indefinable, ineffable, nameless, formless, uncaused, eternal, limitless absolute, without beginning or end. You can experience it—through meditation. And it's definitely worth finding.

What's it like to experience the absolute? Here's how Cliff Waldman, an engineer from Boston, Massachusetts, described his meditation experience:

> "The most complete state of peace and utter contentment I've ever known. It was absolutely perfect, in a bubble of bliss. I had no worries or cares, fear or doubt, no joy or sorrow. In fact, I had no feelings at all. It was different from any normal experience. It felt like everything and nothing, like I was everywhere and nowhere, like I was not this and not that. I was utterly perfect and one with everything. All was right with myself. There was no desire other than to just be."

Usually such a state doesn't last long, particularly in the beginning stages of meditation. We glimpse the absolute for only a moment and often don't notice the experience until it's gone. We go deep within and lose all awareness of body and surroundings. Then suddenly we're back, but while coming back, we feel a surge of radiant bliss and love.

Then we wonder, what happened? Where was I? I was in complete contentment and peace, oneness and wholeness. I had the direct experience of who I AM. And who AM I? Radiant light, love, perfection, a divine being of great power and energy, limitless and unbounded.

Now do you understand how meditation can improve your self-image? Do you see that meditation might, just might, have the power to change a lot of negative programming from your upbringing? Do you realize how self-doubt, unworthiness, and fear can be banished with just a little meditation?

Uncovering Dimensions of Your Self

Absolute pure consciousness, at the core of your being, is the basis of your life and all life in the universe. In individual life, the absolute is called *Atman*. In the life of the universe, it's called *Brahman*. So the deepest part of who you are is the absolute. But other aspects of your higher self exist also.

You're a multi-dimensional, multi-faceted being. Your life is like a building, with the absolute as a foundation. Then layer upon layer of concrete, wood, steel, bricks, and mortar make up the building. These layers represent various bodies.

Surprisingly, your physical body isn't your only body. On higher dimensions you have a mental body, emotional body, and many other subtle bodies that comprise your higher self. You might not be able to see these in the mirror, but they definitely exist. They're invisible to your physical eye, but visible to your inner eye.

Just as in the spectrum of light you see the colors of the rainbow, yet ultraviolet and infrared light are invisible, similarly, the light body that pervades and surrounds your physical body is invisible without clairvoyance—the ability to see with the subtle sense of sight.

Perhaps you've heard of Kirlian photography, which claims to photograph your "aura," the energy field around your physical body. Whether or not Kirlian photographs are genuine, talented clairvoyants can see colors or waves of energy around people, plants, and animals. Some experts can interpret their visions and even diagnose disease. Medical clairvoyancy is a new profession that's gaining a degree of credibility today.

To further clarify the aspects of your inner and outer life, please refer to the chart, "Experiencing Dimensions of Your Self." Basically, your life consists of environment, body, mind, and Spirit, with many layers within

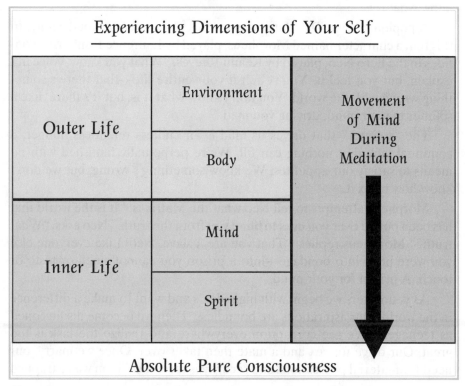

Experiencing Dimensions of Your Self

Outer Life	Environment	Movement of Mind During Meditation
	Body	
Inner Life	Mind	
	Spirit	

Absolute Pure Consciousness

Figure 3a.

those broad categories. Your mind is in constant motion. Meditation is no exception. During meditation your mind moves through all the layers of life, from your outer life, depicted on the upper part of the chart, to your inner life, on the lower part of the chart, until you travel beyond the edge of the chart and experience the absolute, unbounded awareness, beyond all limits of relativity. You transcend the world of duality and embrace the unembraceable, without light or substance, invisible, ineffable, and inexpressible.

A Splinter in Your Mind

How does meditation take your mind through these layers of awareness? Probably your normal habit is to seek happiness in the outer world. You're busy enjoying the pleasures of sensory experience. Yet, no matter how much you seek, no matter how much stuff you buy, or pleasures you get, or power you attain, still your mind is dissatisfied. That's because there's something in the back of your mind. Something you want. But you don't know what it is.

A popular movie *The Matrix* depicts this phenomenon wonderfully. In this film a character named Morpheus, played by Laurence Fishburne, confides in the hero Neo, played by Keanu Reeves, "What you know, you can't explain, but you feel it. You've felt it your entire life—that there's something wrong with the world. You don't know what it is, but it's there, like a splinter in your mind, driving you mad."[1]

The "splinter" that drives us mad is an endless relentless hunger, a continual lack that nothing can fill. We're perpetually famished with no means to satisfy our appetites. We know something's wrong, but we don't know how to fix it.

Morpheus attempts to tell Neo what the Matrix is: "It is the world that has been pulled over you eyes to blind you from the truth." Neo asks, "What truth?" Morpheus replies, "That you are a slave, Neo. Like everyone else you were born into bondage—into a prison you cannot smell or taste or touch. A prison for your mind."[2]

As youngsters we begin with high ideals and want to make a difference in the world. Our aspirations are boundless. Then we become disillusioned as teenagers. We see corruption everywhere and realize the task is too great. Our drive for sex and a mate then takes over. Once we marry, our need for material possessions and security is foremost. Soon we're trapped in a treadmill of endless responsibilities. Work and business consume us. After decades of exhaustion, finally the children are grown and we can retire. By then, we're too weary to enjoy whatever wealth we've amassed. Meanwhile, we have given up our dreams and ideals, and settled for the illusion of security, along with tedium, boredom, and dissatisfaction. A loveless lack-luster life was lived in the slavery of illusion. Thoreau describes this as a life of "quiet desperation."

The splinter in your mind serves a wonderful purpose: It prods you to remove it. It helps you realize there's more to life than you've been living. Happily, that splinter can be removed. Once you realize that what you've been seeking is the one who's seeking, then you can make progress on your spiritual path and free yourself from bondage. The masters of the Far East have tweezers to remove that splinter, a cure for the disease of incessant need. What's that cure? That's right—meditation.

Why does meditation satisfy the perpetual hunger that defines our human condition? Meditation takes you deep within, to the source of satisfaction— the ultimate truth of absolute bliss consciousness, also known as *satchitananda* in Sanskrit. *(Sat:* absolute, *ananda:* bliss, *chit:* consciousness)

In India there's a saying that your mind is like a monkey, jumping from branch to branch. (There are lots of monkeys in India.) Or like a honeybee flitting from flower to flower. My guru used to say that when the honeybee finds a flower with sweet nectar, it will stay still. Similarly, your mind will be satisfied when it experiences perfection at the center of your being— absolute bliss consciousness.

The trouble is—How to find this place? How to locate the nectar?

Just like a honeybee, your senses, endlessly seeking in the outer world, take you far away from the absolute. But by relaxing, settling your body and quieting your mind, you take a 180 degree turn inward. That's how to get where you want to go. By reversing your habit of seeking outward for satisfaction and instead turning within, you'll find genuine satisfaction, the only true satisfaction—eternal bliss consciousness.

A Road Map to Your Inner Life

Look at the chart "Road Map to Your Inner Life" on pages 48 and 49. This chart shows both your gross physical body and many subtle bodies comprising your higher self. Since the chart is quite complex, it can best be understood by experiencing these many dimensions during meditation. This chart provides a complete user-friendly guide to your inner and outer life.

Road Map to Your Inner life

		Faculties	Embodiments	Motives
Outer World (Material World)	Body	1. Earth 2. Water 3. Fire 4. Air 5. Ether	**Environment**	1. Projection 2. Creativity 3. Movement 4. Control 5. Competition 6. Relationship
		1. Smell 2. Taste 3. Seeing 4. Feeling 5. Hearing	**Physical Body**	1. Endurance 2. Survival 3. Propagation 4. Experience 5. Instinct 6. Sensation
	Mind	1. Analysis 2. Assessment 3. Inference 4. Cognition 5. Visualization	**Conscious Mind**	1. Attention 2. Recognition 3. Expression 4. Learning 5. Desire 6. Will 7. Choice 8. Decision
		1. Conditioning 2. Habit patterns 3. Beliefs 4. Memories 5. Ego-identity	**Subconscious Mind (Façade)**	1. Defense, security 2. Status, prestige 3. Accumulation 4. Being admired 5. Being right 6. Power 7. Influence 8. Ownership
		1. Emotions 2. Pleasure and pain 3. Instincts 4. Desires and wishes 5. Moods	**Subconscious Mind (Feeling)**	1. Need 2. Attachment 3. Conditional love 4. Fleeting joy 5. Resentment 6. Anger 7. Pain 8. Fear 9. Guilt 10. Sadness

Façade Barrier (False Belief in Separation from God)

Road Map to Your Inner life (continued)

		Faculties	Embodiments	Motives
Inner World (Spiritual World)	Mind	1. Clairvoyance 2. Clairaudience 3. Clairsentience 4. Intuition 5. Immortality	Etheric (Soul) Self	1. True desires and purpose 2. True identity and expression 3. Freedom of choice 4. Joy and freedom 5. Continuity and purity
		1. Divine love, joy 2. Divine light, lifting 3. Healing, teaching 4. Comfort, peace 5. Salvation, protection	Christ Self	1. Inner guidance 2. Blessing and healing 3. Unconditional love 4. Protecting and comforting 5. Redeeming and forgiving
	Spirit	1. Existence, being 2. Awareness 3. Truth, wisdom 4. Knowing, teaching 5. Serenity, protection	"I AM" Self	1. Strength, authority, and dominion 2. Knowing "I AM that I AM" 3. Tranquility and beingness 4. Realizing inner truth 5. Expressing divine destiny
		1. God-presence, power 2. Glory, splendor 3. Bliss 4. Holiness 5. Oneness, wholeness	God Self	1. Sanctification 2. Being one with Spirit 3. Unification with God 4. Devotion and surrender 5. Infinite light and love
		1. Unboundedness 2. Omniscience 3. Omnipotence 4. Infinity, eternity 5. Cosmic, galactic	Cosmic Self	1. Expansion 2. All-pervasiveness 3. Embodying the cosmos 4. Universality 5. Permanence
	Present Everywhere	1. Formless, nameless 2. Transcendental 3. Attributeless 4. Indivisible 5. Eternal bliss	Absolute Pure Consciousness	1. Perfection everywhere now 2. Equilibrium and balance 3. Peace and harmony 4. Radiance and enlightenment 5. Uninvolved witness of creation

Figure 3b.

When you follow such a road map, you won't get lost, or stumble into any pitfalls along the way.

In this chart both your outer material life and your inner spiritual life are depicted. Your outer life consists of your physical body and mind. Your inner life contains a deeper part of your mind, known as your soul self, as well as many layers of Spirit. A dotted line separating your inner life from your outer life is called the façade barrier. This façade or false mask not only prevents you from knowing who you are, but also isolates you from Spirit.

As you discovered earlier in this chapter, you're a multi-dimensional being. The ovals running down the middle of the chart depict a few of the many subtle bodies that comprise your aura (energy field). Beyond all these aspects of your higher self, the absolute pure consciousness is shown at the bottom of the chart.

The faculties and motives of each of the embodiments are listed beside the ovals. This chart is so detailed that it requires very little explanation. By studying it, and my book, *Divine Revelation*, you'll open your eyes to new dimensions of your self that you never knew existed.

When you look at this chart, don't you feel like knowing more about these levels of identity? Aren't you inspired to dive deep within and experience higher aspects of your being? Meditation is the way to experience everything shown on this chart. And much more.

So many rich experiences await you in the realms of Spirit, so many rewarding avenues to stroll down. As you open to Spirit, you will find exciting new adventures around each bend. Your higher self will guide you to amazing travels, as long as you're open to uncovering the mysteries of the journey.

In this book you'll learn to open your heart, mind, and soul to the riches of inner divine contact. Through meditation, you won't just study this chart; you'll experience it yourself. For this chart isn't just an intellectual exercise. It can help you realize your higher self in a profound and mystical way—through direct experience.

Meditation is a deep way to know yourself. I daresay it's one of the best ways. Certainly, the easiest way. The next section of this book is dedicated to helping you learn how to meditate the easy way.

"What we are looking for is what is looking."
—St. Francis of Assisi

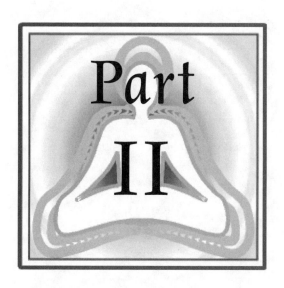

Part II

Discovering
Meditation

Chapter 4

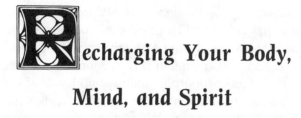echarging Your Body,

Mind, and Spirit

In This Chapter:
- Advantages of Meditation.
- Dispelling Meditation Myth.

Chapter Affirmation:
"I AM the resurrection and the life."
　　　　　　　—John 11:25

Pick up any newspaper or turn on the television. What do you see? Every variety of misery in the form of disease, violence, lack, poverty, oppression, bigotry, hatred, environmental pollution, and other manifestations of fear. All matters of torture justified by the self-righteous. Philosophy, religion, or political opinions shoved down people's throats. People are suffering everywhere. Few appear happy.

Meditation promises a solution to our human dilemma. It offers a way to live in divine harmony, in tune with the laws of nature. Perhaps you think it's naïve to imagine the world's problems solved by meditation. How could sitting in silence transform the planet? Don't we need legislation, treaties, and ambassadors?

It *is* naïve to think meditation can be legislated or forced on people. However, if enough people were to meditate voluntarily, the entire atmosphere of this planet would transform from violence and chaos to peace and harmony. It's a simple function of mathematics:

Meditation is like the "hundredth monkey effect," which you may have read about in Ken Keyes, Jr.'s book by the same title. When a high enough percentage of Japanese monkeys on one island learned to wash their sweet potatoes, monkeys on other islands performed the same task simultaneously.

Rupert Sheldrake, author of *A New Science of Life: The Hypothesis of Morphic Resonance* and *The Presence of the Past: Morphic Resonance & the Habits of Nature,* has developed theories of morphogenetic fields (invisible fields where influences travel) and formative causation (how these fields affect living organisms) that explain this phenomenon. According to his theories, natural systems or morphic units, at all levels of complexity, are animated, organized, and coordinated by morphic fields, which contain an inherent memory. Natural systems inherit this collective memory from all previous things of their kind by a process called morphic resonance, with the result that patterns of development and behavior become increasingly habitual through repetition.

Taking the theory of morphogenetic fields a step further, you might imagine that a high enough percentage of people meditating, with peaceful vibrations in their minds, automatically radiating harmony into the atmosphere, could tip the scales from disharmony to harmony on this planet. Sound strange? Just take a look at the next section. This end result of meditation, along with many other positive results, have been studied scientifically!

Why Meditate?

Over 500 scientific studies have shown how meditation can improve your life and, surprisingly, also transform the atmosphere and potentially improve society. Here are some findings about one effective form of meditation, Transcendental Meditation. All these beneficial results are free from risks, harmful side effects, or adverse reactions, and more cost-effective than medication:

- Reduced violence, crime, accidents, disease, and suicides in populations where a higher percent of the population meditates.

- Beneficial physiological changes during meditation, including reduced metabolic activity, increased brain orderliness and integration indicated by EEG, and increased cerebral blood flow.

- Indicators of reduced stress, such as increased skin resistance, reduced plasma cortisol, reduced arterial blood lactate, and improved muscle tone.

- Reduced hypertension. Improved exercise tolerance and more oxygenation of the heart muscle in coronary patients.

- Reduced risk factors for disease, fewer doctor and hospital visits, reduced health care and medical costs, and less need for medication.
- Improved airway resistance and reduced symptoms in asthmatic patients.
- Reduced insomnia and improved quality of sleep.
- Better periodontal health.
- Less detrimental effects of aging. More factors contributing to longevity.
- Biological age younger than chronological age.
- Higher levels of dehydroepiandrosterone sulfate (DHEA-S).
- Lower average erythrocyte (red blood cell) sedimentation rate (ESR), which is a test that can help determine the progress of certain inflammatory diseases, such as rheumatoid arthritis.
- Reduced psychological distress. Reduced psychiatric hospital admissions.
- Increased self-actualization, mental health, and personal development.
- A more stable, balanced, and resilient personality, emotional maturity, and a positive perspective.
- Reduced use of cigarettes, alcohol, and non-prescribed drugs.
- Better perceptual-motor performance, perceptual acuity, mind-body coordination, and spinal reflex efficiency.
- Increased creativity and intelligence.
- Improved academic performance, moral maturity, orientation towards positive values, and social maturity in college students.
- Better marital satisfaction and adjustment.
- Improved job satisfaction, employee effectiveness, and work relationships.
- Marked improvements in corporate health and performance.
- Greater rehabilitation of criminal offenders and reduced rate of recidivism.

Letting Go of Meditation Myths

Isn't meditation for hippies, geeks, and weirdos who sell flowers at the airport? Isn't it a cult? This is what your rational mind might be saying. After all, it's not the most "normal" activity in the United States heartland. Yet, surprisingly, meditation is practiced in a multitude of forms by millions worldwide.

A certain mystique has developed around meditation. Since it comes from the exotic East, it ain't exactly cornbread, hamburgers, mashed potatoes, chocolate cake, and Coca-Cola. Few people in the Western Hemisphere have any inkling of what meditation is. Many condemn it, even brand it Satanic. Others may have tried it, but gave up long ago, concluding it didn't work. Some stuck their finger into the meditation fire, but got burned, either by a cult, a guru, or due to ignorance, fear, or misunderstanding.

In the mid-twentieth century the word "meditation" was barely in the dictionary. Now it's commonplace. From Transcendental Meditation taught by the Beatles' guru, to Zen meditation, taught by monks in Japan, from subways of New York to sweat lodges of Native Americans, from churches to synagogues, from bedrooms to boardrooms, meditation is practiced in an amazing variety of forms.

Let's examine some meditation myths and overcome any confusion that you might have.

Myth 1: Meditation is for hippies.

If you believe this, then you probably still own a 1969 Chevy. That's how outdated this idea is. In the 1960s, when meditation was first introduced to the West by gurus such as Maharishi Mahesh Yogi, Swami Satchidananda, Yogi Bhajan, Bhagwan Rajneesh, and others, it was practiced by political radicals at the University of California at Berkeley and flower children of the Haight-Ashbury district in San Francisco. But for the past few decades, meditation has spread from the streets of San Francisco to the average Joe's living room, to offices of high-tech companies, influencing all levels of society.

A plethora of meditative practices is found in any given city, from numerous martial arts practices, to Yoga, to Tai Chi, to hypnosis, to Christian centering prayer. Even the most conservative churches offer meditation during their spiritual retreats. Meditative practices are now commonplace in sales, business, and management trainings.

According to statistics in *The Cultural Creatives—How 50 Million People Are Changing the World,* 25 percent of the United States population (approximately 60 million people) regard meditation and spiritual pursuits vitally important and also accept the probability of psychic powers, such as telepathy, knowing the future, communicating with spirits, and so forth. A staggering 61 percent of the population is open to various ways of perceiving and experiencing the sacred in life, believe in psychic and spiritual events, think the divine is both in the world and also transcendent, and believe in developing more awareness.[1] This text goes on to say: "Where the growth rate for the U.S. economy as a whole is two to four percent a year, many of the industries that serve the consciousness movement are growing at 10 to 20 percent a year. The size of the population they serve, and the money involved, is doubling every few years."[2]

Meditation and consciousness expansion is definitely prevalent. It's mainstream. And it's here to stay.

Myth 2: You don't have time to meditate.

The question is not whether you have time meditate, but whether you have time *not* to. That's because your efficiency and success at work, at school, in sports, in society, and in your relationships will increase dramatically when you meditate. Hundreds of studies have demonstrated meditation increases alertness, relaxation, coordination, health, even IQ. It has even been shown to slow down the aging process. With such amazing results, how can you afford not to take time to meditate?

Myth 3: You can't meditate.

Anyone can meditate. Do you have a mind? If you do, then you can meditate. Can you think a thought? If so, you can meditate. Are you alive and breathing, and can you understand simple instructions? Then you can meditate. You can prove it to yourself by using the simple meditation practices in this book.

Myth 4: Meditation is against your religion.

Is there really a religion that's against meditation?

Hindu, Jain, Taoist, Sikh, Confucian, and Buddhist scriptures advocate meditation as a way to attain a state of stillness that reveals the true nature of the self. The Roman Catholic *Spiritual Exercises* of St. Ignatius Loyola and *The Dark Night of the Soul* by St. John of the Cross instruct

Christians to meditate on events of Jesus' life. Christian centering prayer, a form of meditation, is practiced widely today. Sufis meditate on the Qur'an's 99 most beautiful names of God.[3] Jewish mystics meditate on a verse of Torah to uncover its true meaning. Shamanic seekers engage in a vision quest in seclusion to help them break through limitations and discover life purpose. Throughout religious doctrine there are many examples of meditation being advocated:

- King David said, "Commune with your own heart upon your bed, and be silent."[4] "Be still, and know that I am God."[5]

- Isaiah said, "In returning and rest shall ye be saved; in quietness and in confidence shall be your strength."[6]

- Jesus said, "But thou, when thou prayest, enter into thy closet, and when thou hast shut thy door, pray to thy Father which is in secret; and thy Father which seeth in secret shall reward thee openly."[7]

- Mohammed said, "Contemplation for an hour is better than formal worship for sixty years."[8]

- The Sufi 'Ali (Abû Tâlib) said, "Silence is the garden of meditation."[9]

- Lord Buddha said, "Verily, from meditation arises wisdom. Without meditation wisdom wanes."[10]

- Lord Krishna said, "When meditation is mastered, the mind is unwavering like a flame of a lamp in a windless place. In the still mind, in the depths of meditation, the eternal self reveals itself."[11]

- Lao Tzu said, "Attain utmost vacuity; Hold fast to quietude."[12]

- The Sikh Guru Granth Sahib said, "In the cool, dew-drenched night are shining the stars: At this hour are awake the devotees, lovers of God, Meditating each day on the Name—Their hearts meditating on the lotus feet of God, Whom they forsake not for an instant."[13]

- The Jains pray, "As long as I am seated in this meditation, I shall patiently suffer all calamities that might befall me, be they caused by an animal, a human being, or a god."[14]

- Confucius said, "Only after knowing what to abide in can one be calm. Only after having been calm can one be tranquil. Only after having achieved tranquillity can one have peaceful repose. Only after having peaceful repose can one begin to deliberate. Only after deliberation can the end be attained."[15]

If your religious text isn't included in this list, I'll bet the original scriptures of your religion will encourage you to meditate.

So which religion do you belong to?

Myth 5: You're too impatient to meditate.

My guru used to say that the mind always seeks a field of greater happiness. Your mind constantly pursues objects of pleasure that provide more fascination. That's why it continually wanders. It's impossible to keep the mind under control, so there's no point in trying. The reason for impatience is that you want fulfillment now. Experience has proven (and Eastern scriptures say) that the quickest way to complete satisfaction is by reaching absolute bliss consciousness in deep meditation. So why not meditate and enjoy the contentment that you're seeking, right now?

Myth 6: You can't sit still that long.

Although Chapter 5 primarily focuses on a step-by-step method of sitting meditation, there are countless ways to meditate in which you don't have to sit still, or even sit down! Since your higher self is everywhere and every time, you can meditate anywhere, anytime, day or night. You can call upon your higher self while in your car, while walking, jogging, working, speaking, cooking, or studying.

Anytime you call upon the divine presence, anywhere, you'll immediately be filled with divine grace, wisdom, and peace. Let's experiment right now. Take a deep breath. Relax. Take another deep breath. Now call upon your higher self or call upon a sacred name of divinity aloud, and just see what happens. Word your request something like this:

"I call upon ____*(fill in this blank with a sacred name)*____ to be here with me right now, to lift my vibration and to fill me with love, grace, and blessings."

Now close your eyes for a few moments.

Myth 7: You're too tired to meditate.

The issue isn't whether you're too tired to meditate. Rather it's whether you're too tired because you don't meditate. If you *did* meditate, you wouldn't be tired. That's because meditation supplies abundant energy and relieves all tiredness. The source of your being is a fountainhead of unlimited power and vitality. When you meditate and reach that inner wellspring, you can drink your fill. Once you have drunk, that well remains ever brimful.

Myth 8: You're too old to meditate.

The problem here isn't whether you're too old. Instead it's whether you can afford *not* to meditate at your age. With each passing day you're either cheating death or else taking a step closer to the grave. Meditation helps you reverse those steps and become more youthful. Many people have managed to turn back the dial on their biological clocks through meditation.

Myth 9: You can't meditate because you don't believe in God.

Why should you believe in God? After all, how can you believe in something you've never experienced firsthand? In order to have faith, first you need direct experience. Meditation is a way to experience your higher self. You may not have that experience the first time you meditate, but, if you continue meditating, you will. No faith or belief is required. All you need is willingness to learn. The meditation techniques offered in this book are simple step-by-step procedures without dogma, creed, or doctrine. Think of meditation as a science, a science of mind, if you will. It's a way to explore the recesses of your inner being. Like the explorers who traverse outer space, you're a trailblazer into inner space. So put on your inner-space helmet and come with me into the adventure of a lifetime, a divine pilgrimage into the reaches of your higher self.

In the next chapter we'll get started. Let's go!

> *"Meditation is not a means to an end. It is both the means and the end."*
>
> —J. Krishnamurti

Chapter 5

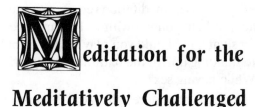

Meditation for the
Meditatively Challenged

In This Chapter:
- Getting Ready to Meditate.
- A Step-by-step Meditation Guide.

Chapter Affirmation:
"I AM the divine indwelling presence."

I s meditation difficult? Does it require discipline, sacrifice, and effort? Many spiritual leaders would have you believe so. They say spiritual progress can only be achieved by abandoning the world, taking up residence in a cave, perched on a deerskin for decades, far away from society and its "evils."

Yet millions of people have proven meditation can be skillfully done by anyone, anywhere, anytime, without any particular belief, lifestyle, habit, or religion. Business people, mothers, teachers, scientists, prisoners, teenagers—people of all backgrounds and professions have meditated successfully. People of nearly all nationalities, political beliefs, races, and religious persuasions are meditating right now.

In this chapter you're going to learn how to do it. Yes. How to meditate, right now. You might think you're incapable, not good enough, not subtle enough, not intuitive enough, not spiritual, any number of "knots." Perhaps you think your wife or sister or pastor can meditate, but not you.

Doubt and fear can be paralyzing when we try something new. But, like any other worthwhile endeavor, meditation is definitely worth taking the risk.

Are You Ready?

Just like other enterprises, meditation requires preparation. You might need a few pointers to help you get with it. For instance, how should you sit—or should you sit at all? Should you play music? Should you lie down? Can you meditate standing up? In the bathtub? When driving a car? While playing tennis? While having sex?

Don't laugh. These questions are valid. And the answer to most of them can be summed up in one phrase: Do what helps you get relaxed and comfortable.

Meditation isn't just for Yogis in pretzel positions or monks who sit rigid while their master whacks them across the shoulders. Meditation isn't performed with clenched teeth and locked jaw. In fact, it's exactly the opposite. It's a way to experience a squishy, fluffy, gushy, mushy state of awareness. Yes, you really did read that. You can even read it again. Squishy, fluffy, gushy, mushy. That's what meditation is—the most fun you can have with your eyes closed and your clothes on. Getting so relaxed, so utterly mellow, like being caressed by hands of such exquisite love and tenderness that you want to weep for joy.

Sounds cool, huh?

So how do you prepare to meditate? First of all, if you're going to take time out of your busy schedule to achieve a deep state of meditation, then make sure you won't be interrupted.

If a flock of three year olds is screaming, raging through your house, maybe that isn't the best time to meditate. Get a baby-sitter to help you have some quiet time to yourself. If co-workers are barging into your office incessantly, it's not the best place to meditate. That is, until you post a sign on your door: "Do Not Disturb." If your spouse wants your attention, simply say, "Honey, I'll be in a much better mood, and more receptive to you, after I meditate. So just give me 15 or 20 minutes."

In other words, find time and a quiet place to embark on inner exploration. Some people like to meditate in nature. I personally prefer a secure place indoors, a controlled environment without insects, animals, wind, rain, cold, heat, noise, people, or interruptions. Indoors, you can set the temperature, wrap up in your favorite afghan, fluff up your comfiest pillow, turn off the television, prop up your feet, light your favorite candle, burn your favorite incense, or whatever you like. The key, operative expression in this equation: BE COMFORTABLE AND RELAXED.

Ignore those so-called spiritual teachers who claim you must sit on the floor, without back support, in lotus posture, with erect spine, staring cross-eyed. Does that sound relaxed or comfortable? Maybe to some people, but not me. I don't like pain, and I don't think pain enhances deep relaxation.

In any case, the way you sit isn't important. The intention with which you sit is what's important. Why is intention important in meditation? Actually, intention is essential in every endeavor. That's because of a powerful gift given to you by your Creator: free will.

Since you're the author of your destiny, when you set an intention, you're well on your way to fulfilling it. So a powerful meditation goal will serve you well. An intention to experience pure consciousness, the state of *satchitananda,* is a worthwhile goal. Physical, mental, or emotional healing is an excellent aspiration. To know the divine, to converse with Spirit, achieve inner peace, answer a question, solve a problem, or receive creative inspiration—these are all superb meditation goals. Really, your imagination is the only thing limiting what intention you conceive.

So you've got a comfortable, safe, and secure place. You're not going to be disturbed. You've decided on an intention or a goal for your meditation. What's next?

The Do-Nothing Way to Meditate

1. Set a goal.

2. Take deep breaths.

3. Protect and heal.

4. Move inward.

5. Sit in silence.

6. Ask for wisdom.

7. Receive revelation.

8. Give thanks and return.

Figure 5a.

Eight Easy Steps to Deep Meditation

Let's learn an easy eight-step program, a way you can meditate right now.

Step 1: Set a Goal

Say a prayer or an affirmation and state your meditation intention out loud.

Some people think it's enough to just sit down, close their eyes, and begin meditating. I guarantee if those people would start with a prayer, their meditations would improve dramatically. That's because prayer works—so well, in fact, that it's proven scientifically!

The most dramatic scientific research on prayer was done by Spindrift, a sort of Christian Science splinter group, who prayed for yeast cells to grow hearty while a control group of yeast cells were not prayed for. The prayed-for yeast cells showed astounding growth. Why is this significant? Because, this experiment can't be influenced by a placebo effect. In other words, little yeasties don't have brains, so they can't imagine themselves growing or not growing. Therefore the effect of prayer upon the yeast cultures could easily be isolated.

Since you probably have more brains than a yeast cell, you can easily set a meditation goal. By using a prayer of your choice, you can state a powerful goal that will carry your meditation to a wonderful completion.

What follows is an example of a statement that you might use to begin a meditation. Say something like this aloud, or record an audiotape or CD and listen to that recording to guide yourself into meditation. When making a recording, read aloud only the statements in quotation marks:

"I recognize there is one power and one presence in the universe and in my life now—the divine presence. I am one with the power, the light, love, peace, joy, and purity of this holy presence now. I am one with the truth of my being, with the light of the divine—one with wholeness, oneness, and wisdom. I therefore claim for myself the perfect meditation now that proceeds perfectly with divine order and timing. I know that during this meditation I receive spiritual awakening, as much as I can comfortably enjoy. I receive clear, direct, divine contact and communication. I receive divine love and healing. I receive clear, precise answers to my questions from Spirit. I experience the profound reality of absolute bliss consciousness within. The goal of this meditation today is___*(state your goal here)*___. I receive all that is wise for me to receive in this meditation, all this and better. Thank you God and SO IT IS."

You can read the above statement before meditation. Or use any prayer, affirmation, or statement of a meditation goal, preferably something soulful and heartfelt that occurs to you when you sit to meditate. These statements don't have to be formal or sound like prayer. Just simple and clear.

Step 2: Take Deep Breaths
Close your eyes, if you haven't already done so, and take a few deep breaths.

Why is closing eyes important? Because it takes attention away from the environment, with all its fascinating colors, lights, and shapes. Closing eyes turns your attention within. Like a turtle drawing into its shell, your five senses draw inward. To focus on the internal, withdraw from the external. That's meditation.

By taking a few deep breaths, your body immediately relaxes. Do an experiment. Sit comfortably, put this book aside, close your eyes, and take three to five slow, deep breaths. Then open your eyes slowly. Do it now.

Relaxing your breathing is amazing, isn't it? Breath is the key to life. It regulates your energy and sense of well being. Each breath is a gift from Spirit. The word 'Spirit' comes from the Latin root spiritus: "to breathe." By breathing deeply, you can become more vital and energetic. Deep breathing invites Spirit to fill you with joy, peace, love, and harmony. (More about this in Chapter 9.)

Remember to take extremely deep breaths as you go into meditation. Every deep breath takes you deeper. Deep breathing is the single most important key to moving into a profound meditative state.

Step 3: Protect and Heal
Close off your aura and heal internal and external negative influences.

Before you move into deep meditation, ask for divine protection and clear any blockages preventing you from experiencing the true nature of your being. These impediments might be internal or external obstacles, either mental or environmental.

Here are a few affirmations to help you become more attuned to Spirit. Speak these statements aloud, or something similar, before you go into deep meditation. Or you may read these statements onto your audiotape or CD:

"I AM in control. I AM the only authority in my life. I AM divinely protected by the light of my being. I close off my aura and body of light to all but my own divine self.

"I invoke the divine presence to help me eliminate negations and limitations that prevent me from a deep experience of meditation. I now dispel all negations of _____ *(list negative emotions you want to release here)* _____ and all other thoughts and emotions that do not reflect divine light. Instead I now welcome feelings of *(list positive emotions you want to accept here)* _____. I AM now in control. I thank God, AND SO IT IS.

"I heal any interfering beings from the astral plane who might be blocking this process of meditation now. Beloved ones, you are unified with the truth of your being. You are lifted in divine love. You are forgiven of all guilt and shame. You are healed, loosed, and released from loss, pain, confusion and fear. Divine love and divine light fill and surround you now. Attachment to the earth no longer binds you. You are free to go into the divine light now, dear ones. Go now in peace and love.

"I call upon the divine to cut any and all psychic ties, cords, connections, and karmic bonds between myself and any person, place, thing, organization, situation, circumstance, memory, or experience that prevents me from going deep in meditation. These psychic bonds are now lovingly cut, lifted, loved, healed, released, and let go, into the light of divine love and truth. Thank you God, AND SO IT IS."

Step 4: Move Inward

Move step-by-step into deeper dimensions of your self.

Refer to the chart on pages 48 and 49, which illustrates various aspects of your inner and outer life. Take yourself on a little journey through the levels depicted by the ovals running down the center of the chart. Simply by acknowledging each level and taking deep breaths between levels, guide yourself into deep meditation. You might say something like the following aloud, or make a tape or CD and then listen to that recording:

"I now relax the mind and let go of the environment. Any sounds around me only serve to take me deeper into meditation. I release, loose, and let go of all cares and concerns of the day. Whatever limiting thoughts or negative beliefs I have brought with me into this meditation, I give them over to Spirit. I release these limitations and let go of them now as I take a big deep breath...

"I now become aware of my physical body...Anywhere I feel any sensation, tension, or stress, I allow my attention and aware-ness to simply rest on that place or places within the body that need healing. As I place attention on those sensations, I take a few mo-ments of quietude to allow them to dissipate...Now I take a deep breath to go deeper, deeper, into the wells of Spirit...

"I now become aware that the physical body is becoming very relaxed, quiet and still, as the breathing becomes less, the heart rate settles down. Every part of the body is deeply relaxed. I take a big deep breath to now relax the eyes...the forehead...eyebrows...the space between the eyebrows...relax the head, temples...cheeks...the jaw...neck relax...shoulders relax...upper arms, lower arms, relax the hands, the fingers...take another deep breath to relax the chest...the stomach...the upper back, lower back...buttocks, thighs...take a deep breath to relax the knees, the legs, ankles, the feet, toes...the fore-head relax, eyebrows relax...relax the space between the eyebrows. I now take a big deep breath to relax the whole body...And another deep breath to fill up the entire body...Then completely let go and relax...Peace, peace, be still. Be still and be at peace...

"I now become aware of the conscious mind. As I take a deep breath to go deeper...I allow the conscious mind to settle down to complete quietude, just as the body settles to deep relaxation...As the breathing becomes less, the mind becomes quiet. So tranquil and relaxed, like a still pond, without a ripple. The mind rests in deep silence and peace, like the water at the bottom of the ocean, where there is complete calmness, quietude, and serenity. The mind is submerged in that total stillness, at the depth of that silent ocean. As I take a big deep breath to go even deeper into that silence...Peace, peace, be still. Be still and be at peace...

"I now allow the attention to drift into the subconscious realm, where I quietly tiptoe through the maze of the unconscious, leaving untouched anything I might find here. As I move through the sub-conscious mind, my mind settles down to deep peace and relaxation.

I now take a big deep breath and go deeper, deeper, into the wells of Spirit...Peace, peace, be still...

"Now I take a deep breath and walk up to the gate that leads into Spirit. I open the gate quietly...Gliding through the gate, I effortlessly drift over the rainbow bridge that leads into the realm of Spirit...I open my heart to divinity and welcome the holy presence in love. I am cleansed and bathed in the radiant light of the divine. Magnificent streams of heavenly energy vibrate and radiate around me. I bathe in the light of the sacred presence, the holy of holies, the eternal oneness of being, and am exalted at the altar of divinity. I take a deep breath and go deeper, deeper, into the wells of Spirit...Peace, peace, be still...

"I now become aware of the etheric soul self, the perfection of my being, who is magnificent, effulgent, beauteous, filled with splendor and radiance. My eternal soul, ever youthful, joyous, and immortal. I ask the soul self to come forth now and introduce itself to me. I now ask this luminous being to reveal my soul's purpose and true desires...

"Now I take a deep breath and go even deeper, deeper, into relaxation and silence...I go to the level of the Christ self. I ask this brilliant being of golden light to reveal itself to me, that I may recognize the unconditional love, healing, compassion, and salvation of the inner Christ self...

"I take another deep breath...And go deeper into the silence of being, as I call upon the 'I AM' self to come forth now and reveal its splendiferous light of wisdom, beingness, awareness and consciousness. This beautiful, powerful, mighty 'I AM' presence is present here in all its glory...

"As I take another deep breath, I go deeper, deeper, into the wells of Spirit, into the silence of being...I become aware of the God self, with humility, devotion and love, I worship at the altar of inner divinity, which is my higher self. God the good, omnipotent, omnipresent, radiant and filled with light. God is here now and always, at the center of my being...

"I take another deep breath, letting go and letting Spirit take me deeper, deeper still, into the wells of Spirit, to the silence of being...I relax and let go into the cosmic self, which is vast and immense as the entire universe. All the stars, galaxies, and planets, the enormous reaches of the universe are contained within the cosmic self, without limits, unbounded awareness. I now take a deep breath and go deeper...

"As I relax and let go, the conscious mind sinks even deeper, deeper still, into the center of being, into the wells of inner silence. I take a deep breath...As I let go and allow my awareness to touch the breath of the absolute. Beyond the realm of duality, I transcend into the nameless, formless, quality-less, motionless absolute, one without a second, beyond the beyond, absolute _Brahman._ I take a deep breath and ask the divine presence to take me deeper, into the realm of silence, _satchitananda,_ absolute bliss consciousness, at the center of being...I now dwell in that deep silence for some time. If, at any time, I feel like I'm going out of the silence, I take a deep breath to go back in..."

Step 5: Sit in Silence
**Dwell in the silence of the absolute pure
transcendental awareness.**

Once you've attained a state of inner peace and deep relaxation, that's the time to simply let go and remain in quietude. You may stay there for a few seconds, for a minute, or several minutes. There is no time in the timeless. You might notice your awareness resting in _satchitananda,_ the state of _samadhi,_ "Sama" means evenness and "dhi" means intellect. Therefore, "samadhi" means evenness of intellect, or, in other words, equipoise of mind and stillness of body.

Your breathing may become quiet and still, until you're barely breathing at all. Your heart might slow down. Your body might feel numb, transparent, or even vanished. Deeply absorbed in your higher self, you forget body and surroundings. You might not feel deep, but if a phone or doorbell rang, you would realize how deep you were (that is, right after you jump back into your skin, which you just jumped out of).

Step 6: Ask for Wisdom
**Call upon your higher self to answer questions or
give you a message.**

Now the fun begins. Once you're in a deep state of silence, contentment, and inner peace, you can call upon a deity, a divine being, or an aspect of your higher self to come forth and communicate with you. Now you can have conversations with God, in whatever form you believe God to be. You might say something like this:

"I now call upon the divine presence, my higher self, to come forth and bring me highest wisdom for today. Please give me a message that will deepen my inner contact with the divine, uplift me, heal me, and bring forth divine inspiration and joy. I now take a big deep breath and go deep within, into the silence of my being."

The preceding statement is highly general, but you could also ask specific questions of your higher self, such as:

- What would be wise to do about my child's drug problem?
- How can I heal my chronic back pain?
- Please, give me ideas about how to promote my business.
- Is it wise to enter into this particular business partnership?
- How can I find my perfect mate?

Also, you can be specific about which aspect of your higher self you wish to communicate with by calling upon a sacred name. Be sure you don't ask predictive or fortune-telling questions. Otherwise, you'll degrade your meditation into a lower vibration by inviting lower energies to answer.

Step 7: Receive Revelation

Get quiet and still, and wait for the answers to be revealed to you.

Now that you've asked, it's time to receive. So take some deep breaths, get quiet and still. This is the time to practice the do-nothing program: Do nothing, nothing, and less than nothing. Allow your higher self to speak to you. You'll receive the message as a vision, voice, or feeling. These are the three main ways Spirit speaks to you.

You might get a clairvoyant vision, like a motion picture, in your inner eye. Or you may hear inspiring words clairaudiently in your mind or heart. This will sound like any other thought passing through your mind. But these loving, wise words will speak from a deeper source, from the divine presence. Or you may get a clairsentient feeling; a sensing that gives you the message or answers your question.

Whatever you get, most likely it's a genuine message from your higher self. If you have doubts, then put it on the shelf for awhile. Maybe it's a clear revelation, or perhaps your subconscious mind or another influence is clouding the true message. In order to test the validity of inner messages see Chapter 14.

Step 8: Give Thanks and Return

Give gratitude and come back out of meditation step by step.

Now that you've experienced absolute bliss consciousness and you've also experienced your higher self, a deity, or a divine being, it's time to give gratitude and come out of meditation.

To come out of meditation, I recommend you take deep breaths in a specific way. Here's how: Lean forward very slightly in your chair. Now take a big deep breath, and as you exhale, pretend you're quickly, vigorously blowing out a candle. This kind of breath quickly brings you out of meditation into a state of subjective and objective balance. Go ahead and take a deep breath like this right now.

You might say something like the following to bring yourself out of meditation (You can record these statements onto your tape or CD):

"I thank Spirit for this wonderful meditation and for all I have received today. I now come out of meditation step-by-step. I now take a big deep breath and pretend that I'm blowing out a candle...I come forth now, bringing with me all the gifts of Spirit.

"I become aware of the subconscious mind, knowing the subconscious mind has been transformed and lifted by this meditation. The subconscious is now healed of all false habits and conditioning. I heal any limited beliefs, as I let go of the subconscious mind and place it into the hands of Spirit.

"I now take another deep breath and blow out another candle...I become aware of the conscious mind, knowing the conscious mind is conscious of divine Spirit. Conscious mind is one with Spirit, one with the truth of being. The conscious mind is now united with divine mind, and every thought is a divine revelation and inspiration from Spirit.

"I take another big deep breath and blow out another candle...I now become aware of the physical body. This body has been transformed and lifted by this meditation. The physical body is one with the divine body and is transmuted into a radiant body of pure light, brilliance, splendor and magnificence. If it is my choice, the body is becoming an immortal ascension body, youthing day-by-day.

"I take another big deep breath and blow out a candle as I become aware of the environment, yet still keeping my eyes closed...I become aware of my body sitting in the chair, the space around me, coming back to this time and place. I know that I bring into the environment all I have gained from this meditation—all the gifts of Spirit. As I move into daily life I vibrate with the divine presence and radiate it all around me each moment of each day. I am a radiant being of light and messenger of Spirit. I am a walking, talking, breathing, living vessel of the divine, and I realize the magnificence of my inner being. So I let go and allow divine Spirit to guide me in each day.

"I now take four deep vigorous breaths and blow out four candles. Then I come all the way back to objective and subjective balance and then open my eyes . . ."

Speak the following affirmation out loud after opening your eyes:

"I AM alert. I AM awake. I AM objectively and subjectively balanced. I AM in control. I AM the only authority in my life. I AM divinely protected by the light of my being. Thank you God, and SO IT IS."

Do It Now!

You've just learned what I call the Divine Revelation meditation technique. Now is the time to do your own experiment of deep meditation. Either read these statements or make a tape and listen. Go and do it now.

How did it work for you? Did you feel some relaxation or inner peace? If so, your meditation was successful.

If you would like more information on the contents of this chapter and many other chapters of this book, or if you would like to order guided meditation audio or video programs, please see page 254. There you can find detailed information about *Divine Revelation*.

> *"Where there is peace and meditation, then there is neither anxiety nor doubt."*
>
> —St. Francis of Assisi

Chapter 6

ravel Tips for Exploring

Inner Space

In This Chapter:
- Trouble Shooting Meditation Problems.
- Experiencing Higher Consciousness.

Chapter Affirmation:
"I live in the heart of God."

What happens when you run into a meditation problem? Long ago and far away, when meditation students used to live with gurus in *ashrams* (places where gurus live), you could ask your guru questions (if you could travel to India, wait a real long time, get past the guards into your guru's room, and if he was willing to talk to you). Since you probably don't live with a guru, and since you might not be planning to soon, in this chapter let's address some problems or questions you might have. Let's start with questions that might arise about your meditation practice.

FAQ's: Meditation Logistics

Q: What time of day should I sit to meditate?

A: Traditionally, meditation is done at sunrise and sunset. Nature's transition times are optimum periods for spiritual experience, when the

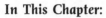

chaos of the day settles to quietude. I recommend meditating in the morning, after bathing and before breakfast. Also, you might meditate again before dinner. Deep meditation is better on an empty stomach, since meditation decreases metabolism, which causes an internal war with food digestion. Also, by meditating too late at night, you might fall asleep and not wake until morning. Or meditation may prevent you from falling asleep. However, you can meditate, or not, whenever you want. Be natural and true to yourself.

Q: How often should I meditate?

A: I suggest you meditate at least once a day. When it comes to meditation, it's a good idea to build up momentum, rather than making a spotty, half-hearted attempt. However, if you don't meditate sometimes, don't beat yourself up.

Q: How long should I meditate?

A: I recommend taking 20 to 30 minutes to meditate. However, you can have a perfectly good meditation in five minutes or 45 minutes. I used to meditate up to 20 hours a day. Yes, you read that right. That wasn't a typo. 20 HOURS a day. But I wouldn't suggest doing more than one hour per day without supervision. Besides, now the planetary vibration has lifted to such a degree that hours of meditation are no longer required in order to achieve deep meditative experiences.

Q: What if the doorbell or phone rings?

A: It's a good idea to decide the answer to this question before you sit to meditate. Then you won't have to deal with the problem in the midst of meditation. Before you ever close your eyes, put a "Do Not Disturb" sign on your door, take the phone off the hook or turn down the ringer and the answering machine, or place someone in charge of handling potential disturbances. Another option is to deal with disturbances as they arise. But if you do, go back and finish your meditation afterward. You might discover it's better to prevent disturbances, because a doorbell or phone ringer can rip you out of deep meditation with a sudden jolt.

Q: What should I do with children, with pets, with my partner?

A: Secure a quiet, sacred space for your "alone time." Tell the kids when they see a sign on your door, "Mommy is Meditating," they must stay downstairs. Pets might jump onto your lap at the most inopportune time, during deep silence of transcendental awareness. So keep dogs and cats downstairs with the kids and meditate undisturbed. If you want your partner to respect your meditation, be sure he/she is informed that you're serious about it. Make meditation a top priority, honor your meditation time as sacred, and treat yourself with respect.

Q: **What if I have to blow my nose, go to the bathroom, scratch, or if my foot falls asleep?**

A: If your nose is running, blow it. If you feel like sneezing, sneeze. If you need to go to the bathroom, get up and go. If you itch, scratch. If your foot falls asleep, move. Simple, natural. Meditation isn't a contest to see how long you can remain motionless. It's a way to relax your mind and body, settle down, and experience the truth of your being.

FAQ's: Unusual Meditation Experiences

Q: **What if I get a strange sensation or experience during meditation?**

A: Please define "strange." Any number of unusual experiences may arise during meditation that never occur during "normal" waking life. You could feel anything from the heights of spiritual elation and supernal bliss to the lows of self-condemnation and negation, which need healing. In any case, your meditation experiences are all natural and from Spirit. Don't doubt them.

Q: **What if I feel like I'm getting lifted or even levitated out of my chair?**

A: A "vibrational lifting" or "quickening" is an experience of consciousness being raised to a higher frequency. Like everything in the universe, you're a vibrational being, composed of energy, light, and space. Meditation attunes you to a higher frequency. Your body-mind vibration might speed up to achieve a new level of awareness. On the spiritual dimensions you can contact your higher self, divine beings, and your subtle bodies, which vibrate at a higher frequency than your physical body.

Q: **What if the experience of lifting is too powerful?**

A: Spirit will never give you more than you can handle. However, if the experiences are too powerful or overwhelming, you can simply say, "Divine presence, please make it gentler."

Q: What if I feel like I'm on fire?

A: The spiritual energy coil *(kundalini)* may rise up your spine (see page 127), which could be perceived as heat or fire. Don't be concerned—there's never been a case of spontaneous combustion during meditation. In fact, "holy fire" is a sign of spiritual attainment. Kundalini rising up the spine and finding blockages along the way may produce heat. Or Spirit might use heat to heal a diseased condition. If heat becomes too intense, just say, "Spirit, please make the experience easier and gentler."

Q: What if power is surging through me?

A: A "power feeding" is great energy coursing through your body. Your body may swell with strength and radiate health and wellness. Often teachers, counselors, or healers are given this extra energy for their spiritual work. Welcome it without resistance. Otherwise it might cause pain. You can say, "I welcome this energy with love and comfort." If the discomfort is too great, say, "Divine presence, please make it less."

Q: What if someone or something is showering love on me?

A: You may receive a "love feeding," a feeling of being loved and nurtured by Spirit. Your heart might open with divine love pouring into or out of it. Your inner teachers, the divine beings around you, may bathe you in divine love and bless you with peace.

Q: What if I feel overwhelmed with joy?

A: Your higher self may give you a "joy feeding." An inner smile might overcome you, seemingly out of nowhere. Divine happiness may well up in your heart and fill your body with bliss. If the feeling of ecstasy becomes uncomfortable, just imagine you're sending this joy out into your environment. This will lessen the intensity.

Q: What if my breathing changes?

A: Your breathing will definitely change during meditation. It will become slower, more regular, quieter, and then finally attain a state of suspension, where breathing becomes imperceptible. In addition, you might receive the "holy breath," spontaneous rapid and somewhat noisy breathing. This blessing from Spirit raises your level of vibration and feeds you divine energy.

Q: What if I see, hear, taste, smell, or feel something unusual?

A: You definitely will, and these experiences are all natural. You might receive a "vibrational signal," a subtle sensory experience that identifies a particular aspect of your higher self.

You might see a particular light of a specific color in a specific place, such as in or near your body. You may see a symbol, such as a rose, a tree, a cross, or a Star of David. A beautiful shimmering angel might appear, or a face of a saint or a deity.

Perhaps you hear beautiful celestial music, harps, humming, an *Om* sound, a tone, rustling leaves, rushing water, or angels singing.

A sweet taste may emerge in the back of your throat or in your mouth when you haven't eaten anything.

You may smell a sweet fragrance of jasmine, sandalwood, rose, lilac, or gardenia when no flower or perfume is nearby.

Energy, heat, tingling, electricity, or other sensations might surge through your body. Something may press on you, surround you, hover near or above you, cloak you, protect you, love you, or feed you energy. Your body may seem a different size or shape, become numb, or disappear altogether.

Your body might shake. Maybe your head moves, rocks, or bobs back, forward, sideways, or in circles. Your eyes might roll back in your head or eyelashes flutter. Your entire body may rock, quiver, move, or vibrate. An extremity might move.

Every one of these experiences is significant and indicates you're in contact with a particular divine being with a specific name. If you get one of these experiences, ask, "Divine presence, please tell me your name." Once you know the name, you can identify that divine being later on by the same signal. More about using signals on page 190.

Q: What if I leave my body?

A: There are several ways to travel to the inner planes. The best way is through etheric projection. Your higher self is already in all places, dimensions, and times. By simply placing attention on a particular place, your awareness can be there instantaneously. Also you can travel to higher dimensions in your *anandamaya kosha* (bliss body: see page 221) or another divine body. Astral projection, on the other hand, means leaving the physical body and traveling to the astral plane in your

pranamaya kosha (astral body: see page 219), which is connected to
the physical body by a silver cord. If you find yourself outside your
body or hovering above it, repeat the self-authority affirmation on
page 155.

Q: **What if I feel like I disappeared?**

A: Congratulations, you've attained the fortunate state of samadhi in
transcendental bliss consciousness, where awareness of body and
surroundings disappears altogether. In that state you're so absorbed
in inner peace and bliss that you forget everything else.

FAQ's: Uncomfortable Meditation Experiences

Q: **What if I fall asleep during meditation?**

A: Sleep is a sign you're meditating successfully. That's because meditation brings deep relaxation. If your body needs sleep, you'll naturally
fall asleep. If you often fall asleep in meditation, here are a few suggestions: Perhaps you're suffering from sleep deprivation. Therefore,
get more sleep at night. If that doesn't work, meditate first thing in
the morning, when you're fresh. Or, if you meditate later in the day,
take a nap before meditating. If you still fall asleep in meditation,
then you need a serious vacation—the kind where you spend most of
your time sleeping.

Q: **What if my mind wanders during meditation?**

A: You aren't unique. Everyone's mind wanders during meditation. The mind is a monkey, swinging to and fro, yapping and
cawing, searching for that ripe banana. That's okay. No problem. There's a reason that I suggest you either speak aloud to
guide yourself into meditation, or use a guided meditation
tape: Your mind won't have a chance to wander far. And it
will have a chance to wander in the right direction: toward
infinite bliss.

Q: **What if something scary happens or I feel I'm getting out of control?**

A: During meditation there's nothing to fear. Allow yourself to be held
in the arms of divine love. If something frightening comes up, then
immediately open your eyes and say the self-authority affirmation on

page 155. Then take a few deep breaths and go back into meditation. If you still feel afraid, then say: "The light of God surrounds me. The love of God enfolds me. The power of God protects me. The presence of God watches over me. Wherever I am, God is, and all is well." Then take a few deep breaths and go back into meditation. If something overwhelmingly frightening happens, then immediately say the astral healing prayer on page 158 in a clear voice. Then take a few deep breaths and go back into meditation. If you're still having problems, then repeat the above process.

Q: What if an uncomfortable feeling or a pain arises in my body?

A: Discomfort or pain during meditation has three possible causes:

1. Your sitting posture is causing discomfort.
2. Your body is being healed, and that healing is causing painful bodily sensations.
3. You have a bodily disease and need medical attention.

If moving your body doesn't alleviate the pain, then, most likely, stress release or deep healing is occurring. Any number of unusual sensations may arise. That's because in meditation the body rests more deeply than sleep. Given the right conditions, the body naturally tends to heal itself. Meditation conditions are optimal for healing. Therefore, uncomfortable sensations often indicate the body is healing.

For example, a software engineer named Tom Hathaway, of San Jose, California, reported, "I went through a week of excruciating meditations, like my leg was being ripped open, torn apart, and put back together again. At the end of the week, my leg, which suffered a serious injury years before, suddenly felt normal, like it did before the injury. I no longer needed my cane. I was thrilled with my higher-self medical-house-calls."

If you get strange sensations during meditation, as my guru used to say, "Take it easy, and take it as it comes." Maybe your Spirit-doctor is making house calls today. But if those pains persist, better see your local M.D.

Q: What if uncomfortable sensations or pains overwhelm me?

A: Pain and discomfort might be so intense that you can't listen to the tape nor do anything else. In such a case, take deep breaths. Then allow your conscious attention to quietly rest on that place or places where you feel those sensations. Don't do anything with the sensations. Don't try to "heal" or manipulate them. Just quietly feel them with a neutral attitude, until they finally lessen or dissipate. Pain is an interesting phenomenon. It's your body's way of begging for attention. Give the body the attention it needs by feeling the sensations; then, most likely they'll change, become less or more, and eventually diffuse.

Q: What if an intense thought or emotion grips me during meditation?

A: Perhaps you're going through tough times. Maybe an overwhelming emotion comes out of nowhere. This can be confusing and disconcerting. In this case, it's better to feel the feelings, without judging them. Let emotions flow. Don't resist or stop them. Allow yourself to get angry or sob. After the emotion has run its course, say the thought-form healing affirmation on page 157. Then take deep breaths and go deeper into meditation. Pretend you're sinking out of your head and into your heart with each exhale.

Attaining Meditation Goals

How to Succeed	How to Fail
1. Allow Spirit to guide you.	1. Float around in daydreams
2. Pray for clarity and divine order.	2. Drift in scattered thinking.
3. Use the power of prayer to heal.	3. Leave your body.
4. Be rested and clear.	4. Go blank or unconscious.

Figure 6a.

FAQ's: Failure to Meditate

Q: What if I feel restless or agitated, can't sit, or can't even get started?

A: Restlessness arises from mental agitation, usually due to hyperactivity. A few ways to calm your mind before meditation are:

1. Take some deep breaths.
2. Take a soothing bath.
3. Take a nap.
4. Pray or say affirmations. Either read the opening prayer on pages 64 and 65, read a prayer from a scripture of your choice, or say healing affirmations in Chapter 11. Prayer soothes and relaxes your mind.

Q: What if I can't relax during meditation?

A: Why do you suppose you aren't relaxed? Is it because you're sitting uncomfortably? If so, get more comfortable. Use more pillows. I don't advise lying down, because you might sleep through meditation. Sit up, but do so in comfort. Are you trying to concentrate? Then stop. Just stop what you're doing. Take a big deep breath. Relax. Meditation is the opposite of strain. It's deep relaxation. Don't try to control your mind or blank it out. It won't work, and you might get a headache. Are you worried and can't let go? Then use the thought-form healing on page 157. Then take deep breaths, and as you breathe out, pretend you're sinking out of your head and into your heart. Let go and let God.

Q: What if I'm afraid to let go?

A: This is a common experience, since many people are taught to maintain a firm grip on their minds at all times. To them, letting go of the mind equates with insanity. Meditation, however, is a normal, natural, safe process. In fact, it's the exact opposite of mental illness. Taking deep breaths will help you relax and let go. As you breathe out, pretend you're sinking into your heart. If you're still afraid, do the thought-form healing on page 157 to heal your fear. If necessary, do the past-life healing on pages 159 and 160.

Q: What if I'm not getting anywhere in meditation?

A: Define what you mean by "not getting anywhere." Where, exactly, do you want to "get"? Meditation is a natural process. You'll get whatever you need in each meditation. It's not a good idea to have particular expectations, to compare meditations of other people with yours, or compare one meditation with another. Every meditation is in divine order and conducted by Spirit. Just trust that Spirit guides you in the most wondrous ways.

Q: What if I find meditation hard to do?

A: It doesn't take rocket science to follow the guided meditation in the previous chapter. The easiest way is to make an audio recording and play it back. Then just follow the simple instructions. Sometimes, when you're listening to the tape, your mind might drift. Then, when you realize you "spaced out," just continue to listen to the tape and follow the instructions, without rewinding the part you missed. It doesn't matter. You get the benefit of meditation, whether your mind wanders or not. If you still find meditation difficult, maybe you're straining to concentrate or control your mind. Maybe you're sitting rigidly. Meditation is supposed to be effortless. It's a way to accomplish everything by doing nothing. Think of meditation as the do-nothing program: Do nothing, nothing, and less than nothing.

Q: What if I don't go deep into meditation?

A: Define "deep." I promise if you take full, deep breaths, and follow the instructions in Chapter 5, you'll get into a state of meditation. Often you don't realize how deep you are, until a loud noise jolts you out of meditation. If you still think you're not "deep," here are some suggestions:

1. Say out loud, "Divine presence, take me deeper into meditation." Then take some deep breaths.

2. With each deep breath, imagine you're sinking out of your head and into your heart.

3. Say the thought-form healing affirmation on page 157. Then take some deep breaths and go deeper.

Q: **What if I don't get a message or an answer to my question?**

A: During meditation your message will most likely be an inner voice, vision, or feeling. If you're not getting the message, you can ask, "Dear divine presence, take me deeper into meditation." Then take some deep breaths and go deeper. As you exhale, sink out of your head and into your heart. Get quiet. Do nothing, nothing, and less than nothing. Take more deep breaths and do even less than that. In that state of inner stillness the message will simply "occur to you" in a gentle, quiet way, like any other thought drifting through your mind.

Your higher self might also give you an answer outside of meditation. Just be receptive. It may come as a dream, visitation, omen, message from a friend, psychic reading, through divination, an "aha" experience, flash of light, coincidental events, déjà vu, dowsing, or muscle-testing. (You can read about 12 ways to receive inner revelation in my book, *Divine Revelation*.)

Q: **What if meditation doesn't work for me or I don't feel motivated?**

A: Record an audiotape or a CD, as recommended in the previous chapter. Follow the instructions. You would feel motivated if you were getting experiences of divine Spirit. If, after attempting the guided meditation several times using your CD or audiotape, you still don't get satisfactory results, then consider taking a meditation class. To find a teacher or order tapes, visit my Web site listed on page 254 or call the phone number listed on the same page.

Q: **What if I'm just not cut out for sitting still in meditation?**

A: There are many ways to meditate other than just sitting still. I recommend reading Paul Reps' book *Zen Flesh, Zen Bones*. In the chapter called "Centering," you can learn 112 ways to experience transcendental awareness, some of which can be practiced during activity.

FAQ's: Problems After Meditation

Q: **What if I feel weird, spaced-out, headachy, disoriented, or discombobulated after meditation?**

A: Strange feelings after meditation indicate you came out too abruptly. Never jump out of meditation, unless it's an emergency, in which case it's imperative to go back, finish your meditation, and come out slowly. If you take enough time and enough deep breaths at the end of meditation, and if you say the affirmation on page 72, then you should have no problems after meditation. Be sure the coming-out-of-meditation breaths are different from the going-into-meditation breaths. At the end of meditation sit up straight or even lean slightly forward, breathe in deeply, and then blow out vigorously, noisily, and quickly, as if you're blowing out a candle.

Q: What if I'm in a bad mood after meditation?

A: You wouldn't be in a bad mood unless: you came out of meditation too quickly, you were straining to control your mind or to concentrate, or during meditation you stayed on the surface level of your mind.

What do I mean by surface level? Your life has many levels, as depicted on the chart on pages 48 and 49. If your mind stays on the conscious or subconscious level during meditation and never goes beyond the façade barrier, then it's like a diver who belly-flops and doesn't go deep into the water. The best divers glide beautifully into the water, barely make a splash, and go deep. Similarly, your meditation is most successful when you dive deep into Spirit. By floating on the surface, you don't accomplish the goal of meditation; namely, to experience the divine presence deep within. Sublime experiences can't be found on the surface. The higher self is on a deeper dimension, which you can attain simply: Take deep breaths. Sink out of your head and into your heart. Do nothing, nothing, and less than nothing. If necessary, use one or more of the healing affirmations in Chapter 11. Then take deep breaths to go deeper.

"Meditation provides a way of learning how to let go."
—John Welwood

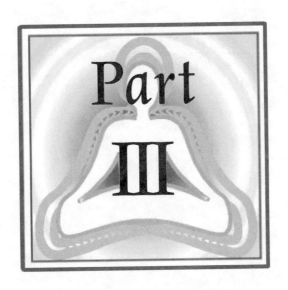

Discovering Yoga

Chapter 7

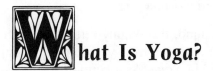

What Is Yoga?

In This Chapter:

- Defining Yoga.
- Introducing Vedic Literature.
- The Paths and Branches of Yoga.

Chapter Affirmation:

"I AM merged, united, and one with Spirit."

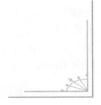

The term *Yoga* is fraught with misconceptions. Usually it's defined as a low-impact exercise program that tones and stretches the muscles. Although the discipline called Hatha Yoga does include specific postures, Yoga doesn't mean exercise. The Sanskrit word comes from a root that signifies, "to yoke." In other words, Yoga means "unity" or "integration." But this unity doesn't refer to union of the nose with the knee or the forehead with the floor. It's supreme union of the individual soul with Spirit—union of individuality with universality.

The state of Yoga can be attained by anyone from any background, not just mystics from the East. Anyone who wants divine contact and divine love, light, power, and energy can experience this. There isn't one sole way to experience Yoga. People from every culture seek unity with the divine, and all religions and spiritual paths have validity.

What Lord Krishna Said about Yoga

Yoga is an ancient philosophy, founded by the sage Patanjali. In the *Bhagavad Gita (Bhagavad:* God, *gita:* song), the most revered scripture of India—the kernel of Eastern philosophy—Lord Krishna, a divine *avatar* (incarnation of God), initiates his disciple Arjuna into mysteries of Yoga. In this dialogue, Lord Krishna says:

> "When the mind, thoroughly settled, is riveted in the higher self, then the person, free from yearning for all enjoyments, is said to be established in Yoga. As a lamp in a windless place does not flicker, such is like the subdued mind of the Yogi absorbed in the self. The state in which the mind finds rest, stilled by the practice of Yoga, is the state that, seeing the self by the self, finds contentment only in the self."[1]

Here Lord Krishna is often misunderstood as advocating austerity and renunciation. But he's actually describing the goal of Yoga—*samadhi* (equanimity of mind and body), the fulfillment of all seeking and source of satisfaction, beyond which no greater enjoyment exists. When you achieve that state, you're free from longing. Your mind is steady, like a "lamp in a windless place" or a honeybee enjoying nectar.

What Yoga Can Do for You

Yoga is a complete science of mind, body and Spirit. Its holistic approach can help you become happier, in tune with natural life, free from habits that cause disease. It heals the body, clarifies the mind, and strengthens the spirit. Studying Yoga can purify and balance your life. It improves health, develops mental concentration, and promotes inner peace.

This book is filled with methods to help you master Yoga (union with divine Spirit). This section of the book focuses on ancient yogic techniques of exercise and breathing. Yoga practices include the following:

1. Yoga *asanas* (physical postures), stretch the muscles, lubricate joints, improve flexibility and posture, increase circulation, enhance concentration, and reverse aging. Also stimulation of acupuncture points increases life energy.

2. *Pranayama* (yogic breathing) awakens the flow of *prana* (Sanskrit) or *chi* (Chinese), the life force, which reverses mental illness and increases alertness, rejuvenation and spiritual awakening.

3. Deep relaxation recharges the body, reduces stress, reverses aging, and improves health. Physical, mental, and spiritual relaxation conserve *prana* (life force in breath).

4. Healthy diet consists of natural organic foods: unprocessed, free from chemicals and pesticides. Such a diet, along with regular fasting, promotes long life, robust health, and disease prevention.

5. Exercise, breathing, relaxation, diet, and positive thinking are just preparations for meditation—the crown jewel of Yoga.

What Is the Veda?

The following section explains where the science of Yoga fits into Indian philosophy. It's not mandatory to study Vedic texts to benefit from Yoga. However, you might be curious to learn more about East Indian philosophy. The *Vedas*, the ancient supreme knowledge of India, began as an oral tradition passed from father to son, chanted generation to generation from time immemorial. The Vedic hymns are said to be vibrations or impulses of sound that underlie, generate, and give rise to the entire universe. The theory is that name is the precursor of form. This is called *nama-rupa* (name and form).

The apostle John said, "In the beginning was the Word, and the Word was with God, and the Word was God."[2] According to Vedic tradition, that "Word" is the primordial seed sound *om,* also known as *pranava.* When this hum stirs, it activates the three gunas, which combine to produce the *mandalas* ("circles": chapters) of the Vedas, which generate all phenomena. (Please refer to page 217.)

In time these oral traditions were transcribed. This Vedic literature is comprised of two branches: *Shruti:* "heard"—divinely revealed hymns, cognized by *rishis* or seers, and *Smriti:* "remembered"—rules, ethics, and moral values for ideal speech, behavior, and health.

Shruti

The Vedas are four in number: *Rig Veda:* wisdom of verses, the oldest Veda, *Sama Veda:* wisdom of chants and melodies, *Yajur Veda:* wisdom of rituals and sacrifices, and *Atharva Veda:* wisdom of priests and magic incantations. These comprise *Samhita:* Vedic *mantras* or *richas* (hymns). Each Veda is chanted in a unique rhythm and meter.

Vedic Literature

	Rig Veda — verses	Sama Veda — chants and melodies	Yajur Veda — rituals and sacrifices	Atharva Veda — priests and magic
SHRUTI (heard) — **Vedic Hymns**				
Vedic Texts	Brahmanas — instructions for yagyas	Aranyakas — forest texts		Upanishads — those who sit near
SMRITI (remembered) — **Vedangas** limbs	Shiksha — sound	Kalpa — timing	Vyakaran — grammar	Nirukta — semantics	Chhandas — meter	Jyotish — astrology
Upangas subordinate limbs	Nyaya 16 — tests of reason	Vaisheshika 9 — elements of universe	Sankhya 25 — elements of human	Yoga 8 — limbs of unity	Karma Mimansa — criteria of action	Vedanta — end of Veda: unity
Upavedas subordinate Vedas	Ayurveda — medicine	Gandharva Veda — music and dance	Dhanura Veda — behavior	Sthapatya Veda — architecture
Puranas story books	Itihash	Ramayana — Story of Lord Rama		
		Mahabharata — Story of "Great India"		

Figure 7a.

Other books classified as Shruti are *Brahmanas:* instructions for Vedic *yagnas* (rituals), *Aranyakas:* "forest texts," mysteries about secret rites for those who live in seclusion, and *Upanishads:* "those who sit near," secret teachings of supreme knowledge given to disciples by spiritual masters.

Smriti

The *Vedangas,* limbs *(anga)* of the Veda, are *Shiksha:* sound, pronunciation, and rhythm of Vedic hymns, *Kalpa:* timing of Vedic rituals, *Vyakaran:* Sanskrit grammar, *Nirukta:* semantics, *Chhandas:* meter, and *Jyotish:* Vedic astrology.

The *Upangas* (subordinate: *upa,* limbs: *anga),* originated by ancient *rishis* (seers) constitute six systems of Indian philosophy, by which the universe is described.

1. *Nyaya,* founded by Gautama, is the science of reasoning, which lists 16 ways to test the procedure for gaining knowledge.

2. *Vaisheshika,* founded by Kanada, offers knowledge of the outer world, and enumerates nine components of the universe.

3. *Sankhya,* founded by Kapila, gives knowledge of the inner world and defines 25 components of the individual.

4. *Yoga,* founded by Patanjali, has eight limbs or branches that unify the outer and inner life in the silence of the self.

5. *Karma Mimansa,* founded by Jaimini, provides criteria to evaluate any action.

6. *Vedanta,* founded by Vyasa, is the end *(anta)* of the Veda, supreme knowledge, where boundaries dissolve into wholeness: non-dualism *(advaita).* Vedanta explains how *Brahman* (the absolute) appears as *Ishwara* (the personal God): The non-dual splits into duality by virtue of *maya* (that which is not, which doesn't exist). Maya's counterpart in the individual, *avidya* (ignorance) causes *atman* (higher self or immortal soul) to appear as *jiva* (individual ego). More about this later.

The *Upavedas,* subordinate *(upa)* Vedas, include *Ayurveda:* science of life *(ayu),* Indian medicine; *Gandharva Veda:* science of music and dance; *Dhanura Veda:* science of behavior; and *Sthapatya Veda:* science of architecture or Indian feng shui.

The *Puranas,* written by Vyasa, bring Vedic knowledge to common people through heroic stories of Gods, sages, seers, and kings. The *Itihash* are two main Puranas, Indian classics of literature called *Ramayana* and *Mahabharata*. The *Bhagavad Gita* is part of the *Mahabharata*.

Eight Paths of Yoga

Yoga philosophy is one of the Upangas, subordinate limbs of the Veda. There are many pathways to Yoga. Eight are briefly described here:

Hatha Yoga: path of physiological culture

Hatha (solar-lunar) *Yoga* is divine union through purifying the body and refining the breath. Every mental state, such as waking, dreaming, or sleeping, has a recognizable physical state. Similarly, higher states of consciousness can be attained through *asanas* (body postures), *pranayama* (breathing exercises), disciplined lifestyle, special diet, and a vigorous elimination program.

Hatha Yoga is suited to those with time and inclination to study diligently in a controlled environment. Hatha Yogis, are naturally reclusive, abstain from food, sex, sleep, and social interaction. Their practices are rigorous and austere.

Raja Yoga: path of mental and sensory control

Raja (royal) *Yoga* uses meditation to develop one-pointed steadiness of mind. Whereas Hatha Yoga controls the mind by culturing the body, Raja Yoga controls the body by subduing modifications of the mind *(chitta vrithri)*. This path uses Mantra Yoga, mentally repeating specific Sanskrit words. Using the subtle sense of hearing, mantras bring the mind to the experience of bliss consciousness, which quiets the mind and controls the senses naturally.

Karma Yoga: path of action

Karma (action) *Yoga* attains union by living according to natural law. In the *Bhagavad Gita*, Lord Krishna said to his disciple Arjuna, *"Yogasthah kuru karmani,"* which means "Perform action established in divine union (Yoga), O Dhananjaya (winner of wealth), renouncing attachment and balanced evenly in success and failure; equilibrium is called Yoga."[3]

This verse means first meditate, then act. It doesn't mean renounce the world and hide in a cave. In deep meditation your mind attains divine union: inner peace, silence, and equanimity. Then, after meditation, still relaxed and settled, act without attachment to rewards, without being affected by or dependent on your environment for fulfillment. Instead, find contentment from the inner fountainhead of joy.

Lord Krishna further elaborates on this point by saying, "You have control over action alone, never over its fruits. Let not the fruits of action be your motive, nor let yourself be attached to inaction"[4] and "Yoga is skill in action" (*Yogah karmasu kaushala*).[5]

By spending a few minutes each day in the state of Yoga, your mind gets saturated with bliss consciousness. Then after meditation, pure awareness naturally gets integrated into everyday life. Karma Yoga is achieved through alternating meditation with dynamic daily activity.

Gyana Yoga: path of knowledge

Gyana (knowledge) *Yoga* removes ignorance by discerning the real from the false, eliminating the veil of illusion, and attaining supreme knowledge. This path must be learned from a realized soul, a teacher who can open your eyes to reality. Through logic, the Gyana Yogi recognizes the following:

1. Relative creation is perishable, futile, and fleeting, bound by space, time, and causation.

2. The universe is *mithya* (phenomenal) and therefore non-existent.

3. The imperishable, eternal, absolute reality, devoid of form and phenomena, underlies creation.

4. The perishable is distinguished from the imperishable.

5. The ultimate truth is "I AM That, thou art That, and all this is That."

6. This reality is assimilated and expressed in everyday life.

No one can define the indefinable ultimate reality. As Lao Tsu said, "The Tao that can be put into words is not the eternal Tao."[6] Therefore Gyana Yoga seeks reality by eliminating everything it's not: *neti, neti* (not this, not this). Since nothing in the phenomenal world is real, this path rejects everything. It eliminates false identifications with body, senses, mind, intellect, will, feelings, and ego, the sense of I-ness. Finally the seeker realizes the seeker seeking the seeker.

Kundalini Yoga: path of prana

Kundalini Yoga, Laya Yoga, or *Kriya Yoga* awakens divine energy in the body through raising *kundalini shakti* (power coiled at the base of the spine like a serpent), upwards through the *chakras* (plexuses of subtle nerve centers).

Kundalini Yoga is an aggressive path of rigorous *asanas* (physical postures), intense *pranayama* (breathing exercises), *bandhas* (muscular locks) *mudras* (gestures), meditation using mantras and imagery, strict dietary and behavioral control. Kundalini flows downward as sexual energy and upward as spiritual energy. Therefore celibacy is essential to this path. (More about kundalini shakti and chakras in Chapter 9.)

The seeker who tries to raise kundalini without the proper guidance of this book or a fully realized master can get into trouble. Frightening experiences, intense physical pain, burning bodily heat, sexual obsession, even mental illness may result.

Bhakti Yoga: path of devotion

Bhakti (devotion) *Yoga* opens the heart of the seeker, bringing direct divine contact through surrender. Divine love develops compassion, charity, and service for God's creatures and God's children. A heart melted in divine love, in remembrance of the divine name, in dedication to the divine presence, attains supreme grace and unity in fullness of joy. Blind faith is the path and fulfillment is the goal. The devotee gets drowned in the ocean of divine love.

Bhaktis are known for unbridled displays of emotion in devotional chanting, singing, dancing, prayer and rituals, and daily conversations with God as an intimate friend or companion.

Although Bhakti is the simplest path, few people have capacity for such deep emotion and one-pointed devotion. But lucky are those who do, since it's a pathway of such utter happiness.

Tantra Yoga: path of fulfillment

Tantra (technique) *Yoga* fulfills desires, solves problems, and achieves results using the intrinsic power of mantras, yantras, and tantras. As mentioned in Chapter 1, a mantra is a name or phrase used as an invocation. A yantra is a geometric representation of a deity, which is drawn, painted, etched, or carved, and then used in ritual, gazed at, or visualized. And a tantra is a specific action to alleviate a problem or achieve a goal. An example: feeding black beans to the needy on Saturdays to ameliorate a problem indicated by the planet Saturn. Sound strange? Perhaps not strange, just foreign to our Western mind.

Tantric *bij* (seed) mantras are powerful sounds with specific vibrational frequencies. Chanting or thinking these potent mantras takes the seeker to higher awareness, generates healing, or elicits particular results. Whereas Vedic mantras are Sanskrit words with specific meanings, Tantric bij mantras are meaningless sounds that invoke particular deities.

Tantrics are like psychologists who dig into our shadow side to unearth innermost fears, cravings, and obsessions. Whereas other paths sublimate instincts, Tantra befriends and embraces them. Once desire exhausts itself, it collapses back to its source: transcendental awareness. Then desire disappears. Those who associate Tantra with sexuality are misinformed. Out of 112 practices in the *Vigyana Bhairava Tantra,* a classic text, only four pertain to sexuality.

Because they are involved in digging deep into psychology and unearthing raw emotions, Tantrics worship Mother Divine, the female aspect of God, in her fiercest aspect: Kali Ma, the slayer of illusion and transmuter of despicable emotions. With grim blue skin and red tongue dangling from her mouth, dripping blood, she dons a necklace of human skulls and dances on Lord Shiva's corpse. Like Kali herself, a practitioner of this path thumbs a Tantric nose at all convention.

Integrated Yoga: path of inclusiveness

Integrated Yoga, the path uniting heart, mind, and will, is beyond sectarianism, philosophies, and techniques. Ecumenical and universal, Integrated Yoga honors all paths and traditions with a wide-angle perspective. Independent thinking, internal reference, spiritual integrity, inner guidance, freedom of choice, regard for humanity—all these characterize Integrated Yoga.

Whereas practitioners of other paths need clear boundaries, limits, prescriptions, and supervision, followers of this path are free spirits. Their decisions are based on intuition.

An unbroken continuum of pure bliss consciousness pervading every particle of your being, in each moment, every day, throughout all states of awareness: waking, dreaming, and sleeping—that's fully integrated Yoga.

Eight Limbs of Yoga

An ancient seer named Patanjali is founder of Yoga philosophy. He wrote the *Yoga Sutras* (threads or aphorisms of divine union) in approximately the second century B.C. The sutras help seekers unify *jivatman* (individual spirit) with *paramatman* (universal spirit).

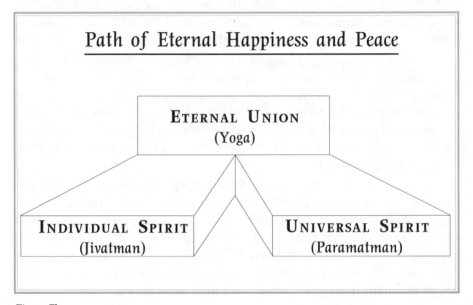

Figure 7b.

Patanjali defines Yoga as "the restraint of the modifications of the mind-stuff *(chitta vrithri)."* He says that once that restraint is accomplished, "then the Seer (higher self) abides in his own nature."[7] Patanjali's *ashtanga Yoga (ashta:* eight, *anga:* limbs) is a description of *kaivalya* (singularity or oneness) and the path to attain it. The following are the eight limbs:

1. Yama: associated with universal life

The first limb of Yoga is *Yama* (abstinence), which upholds the laws of Yoga. The five aspects of yama are:

- *Satya* means truth. The non-changing absolute is eternal truth. A Yogi, therefore, knows truth, lives in truth, and speaks only truth.

- *Ahimsa* signifies non-violence. A Yogi perceives only a state of oneness. Therefore, to harm others would be to harm oneself.

- *Asteya* is non-covetousness. To covet is to possess property that isn't yours. When objects overtake the senses, then those objects possess the self. In contrast, nothing can overtake or possess the self of a Yogi in perfect unity.

- *Brahmacharya* means living *(charya)* the absolute *(Brahman)*. A Yogi dwells in a state of divine unity in perfect contentment. Brahmacharya also signifies conserving sexual energy. Yogis believe preserving sexual fluids transforms these substances into marrow, then blood, then *ojas,* which is the material equivalent of prana (vital energy). Ojas is a sweet, oily, fragrant substance that covers the skin, imparting divine radiance and charisma.

- *Aparigraha* means non-accumulation: freedom from sense objects. A Yogi, ever in unity and wholeness, "content with whatever comes unsought,"[8] seeks nothing from objects of perception.

2. Niyama: link between universal and individual life

Niyama (observance) are laws of Yoga, rules that connect individual life to universal life. There are five:

- *Shaucha* means purity, attained by releasing tension and toxins from the body and false beliefs from the mind.

- *Santosha* is contentment. The only unshakable state of complete fulfillment and satisfaction is absolute pure consciousness.

- *Tapas* ("heat") is abstinence. But it really means senses turn within during meditation, away (abstaining) from sensory objects. The deeper your senses turn within, the more the inner light, the heat of spiritual fervor, glows.

- *Swadhyaya (swa:* self, *adhyaya:* opening the chapter) signifies opening awareness to the self. When the mind turns inward, the chapter of the outer world closes, and the inner world opens.

- *Ishwar-Pranidhan (Ishwar:* divinity, *pranidhan:* bringing into breath) means imbibing the divine when breath is suspended in the state of Yoga. That's surrender to the divine.

3. Asana: associated with body

Asana (seat) indicates stability, to be established in absolute pure consciousness, stable, unshakable—the ultimate state of Yoga. You'll learn some Yoga asanas (postures) in Chapter 8.

4. Pranayama: associated with breath

Prana (life force in breath) and *ayama* (coming and going) indicate movement of breath. Pranayama controls prana, the force of life in breath that harmonizes all movement. A Yogi's breath in transcendental consciousness achieves a state of suspension (More about Pranayama in Chapter 9).

5. Pratyahara: associated with senses

Pratya (direction) and *Ahara* (food) mean introspection: reversing the outward direction of the senses and turning inward, toward ultimate fulfillment. In the Bhagavad Gita, Lord Krishna said to Arjuna, "When, like a tortoise draws in its limbs from all directions, he withdraws his senses from the sense-objects, then the mind of the Yogi is stable."[9]

6. Dharana: associated with mind

Dharana (hold or grasp) signifies the mind held on a fixed point in concentration.

7. Dhyana: associated with intellect

Dhyana (meditation) is flow of the mind in an inward direction.

8. Samadhi: pure consciousness

Sama (evenness) and *dhi* (intellect) signify the state of evenness of mind and stillness of body in transcendental awareness.

Attaining Miraculous Powers

Sage Patanjali's ancient text *Yoga Sutras* explains how enlightenment is achieved through *siddhis* (perfections). Siddhis are supernormal powers acquired by practicing a meditative technique called *sanyama*.

Some siddhis are levitation, walking through walls, lifting unusually heavy weights, disappearing, seeing things at a distance, extra-sensory perception, traveling in a subtle body, making the body very small, large, light or heavy, appearing in physical form in several places at once, walking over water or hot coals, omnipotence, omnipresence, omniscience, and acquiring supreme knowledge.

Patanjali says in the *Yoga Sutras* that three basic elements contribute to mastering the above miraculous powers—intention (dharana), fulfillment (samadhi), and movement between them (dhyana), which unites the first two elements. By using the three elements of dharana, dhyana, and samadhi together in meditation, the siddhi is achieved.

I learned Patanjali's siddhi practice from my East Indian guru, a highly advanced Yogi, with whom I studied for twenty-one years. My experience of sanyama is that it produces divine union, integration, and intense joy. Sanyama can't be taught in a book, but must be learned from a teacher. However, effective methods for meditating as well as for fulfilling your desires can be learned in this book.

> *"Equanimity is yoga. Once one attains that equanimity,*
> *Grace flows continuously."*
>
> —Mata Amritanandamayi

Chapter 8

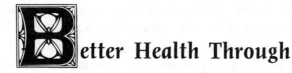

etter Health Through

Yoga Postures

In This Chapter:
- Yoga for Couch Potatoes.
- Practicing Yoga Postures.

Chapter Affirmation:
"I AM perfect health and well-being."

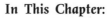

E ven a couch potato can learn the simple Yoga techniques described in this chapter. That's how easy they are. These practices quiet the mind and body and bring attunement to Spirit. Here you'll learn two types of practices: Simple ones, called *Yogic suksma vyayama,* and those that require a little effort, called *Yoga asanas.* The term *asana* means "seat" in Sanskrit. Therefore, rather than Yoga "exercises," they're more aptly defined as poses or postures. Out of 840,000 asanas mentioned in the classic texts of Yoga, only a handful is mentioned here.

As a result of performing these ancient Yoga practices, your body and mind become tranquil and more receptive to the divine presence. But please keep in mind that the exercises and postures in this chapter should be done under the supervision of a qualified teacher and never tried alone without guidance. Consult a qualified medical doctor before attempting any of these exercises, and only do those postures that your doctor recommends.

Getting Ready

The purpose of Yoga asanas is to prepare your mind and body for Yoga—union with the divine. Therefore, do them before meditation rather than after. The best time is in the morning (preferably at dawn), before breakfast, or in the late afternoon before dinner. Your stomach should be empty (four hours since the last food or drink) and bowels cleared. Bathe before asanas or wait at least two hours after asanas before bathing.

Prepare your environment. Traditionally, asanas are done in silence, with focus on body and breathing, without distractions, such as music or television. Also, take time to complete all the postures. Plan to not be interrupted.

Wear loose clothing and be unencumbered. Take off shoes and remove jewelry, necklaces, bracelets, barrettes, and hair bands. Comfort is essential when performing asanas. Cover the hard floor with a couple of thick blankets or an exercise mat. It's best to do asanas near an open window or outside.

Couch-Potato Yoga

Calling all couch potatoes! This is the Yoga for you. These first exercises belong to a category called *Yogic suksma vyayama,* meaning "easy, smallest movement Yoga." These can be done by people of all ages, even the weak, ill, or debilitated. Though simple and requiring little physical effort, these practices produce highly beneficial, profound results.

Unless otherwise stated, these are done in an erect standing position with mouth closed, arms at sides, palms open and fingers together, facing towards your thigh. Breathing is always done through the nose, unless indicated differently. Let's begin.

Prarthana
(Prayer)

Fold hands in prayer with thumbs on the sternal notch (cavity at your throat), and forearms pressed against chest. Close eyes, relax and place attention on your higher power, in whatever form you believe that to be, until you feel a sense of well-being and wholeness. This increases power of concentration and brings communion with higher self.

Udara-Sakti-Vikasaka
(Developing abdominal muscles)

Breathe deeply and quickly through the nose, exhaling and inhaling fully. While inhaling, distend abdomen, and while exhaling, contract it. You may place your hand on your abdomen to make sure you're doing this correctly. Here's a hint: Contract abdominal muscles with a backward push while you quickly, forcefully exhale. Then abdomen will naturally distend during inhalation. During this exercise, inhalation will naturally take longer than exhalation. Repeat at least 10 times. This is also called *Kapalabhati*—breathing like a bellows.

Uccarana-Sthala Tatha Visuddha-Cakra Suddhi
(Clearing the pharynx)

Tilt chin back slightly. Keep eyes wide open and mouth closed. Place full attention on vocal chords (larynx). Inhale and exhale deeply and rapidly into throat like a bellows at least 10 times. This practice clears, dries, and ventilates air passages.

Buddhi Tatha Dhrti-Sakti-Vikasaka
(Developing mind and will power)

Keeping eyes wide open, tilt head back as far as possible. Place full attention on crown of your head. Breathe in and out vigorously through the nose like a bellows at least 10 times.

Smarana-Sakti-Vikasaka
(Developing memory)

Keeping eyes wide open, and head upright, focus eyes on floor at a spot five feet in front of toes. Place full attention on *brahmarandhra* (a point in the brain at the top and middle of your head, about five fingers from hairline) and breathe in and out vigorously like a bellows at least 10 times. This reverses mental fatigue, eliminates nervous exhaustion, and improves memory.

Medha-Sakti-Vikasaka
(Developing intellect)

Close eyes. Lower chin to rest on the sternal notch. This position is called *jalandhara bandha* (chin lock). *Jala* refers to the nerve passing through the neck to the brain. *Dhara* means upward pull. *Bandha* means lock. This bandha creates an upward pull on spinal cord and nerve centers. Place all attention on the depression at nape of neck. Breathe in and out vigorously like a bellows at least 10 times.

Netra-Sakti-Vikasaka
(Improving eyesight)

Eyes open, tilt head back as far as possible. Focus all attention at a spot between the eyebrows with eyes squinted. When eyes feel tired or start watering, then discontinue. This tones and strengthens the eyeballs, cures defective vision, improves visual range, and strengthens concentration.

Karna-Sakti-Vardhaka
(Improving hearing)

Plug ears with your thumbs. Place index fingers lightly on closed eyelids. Close nostrils with middle fingers. Encircle mouth with ring and pinkie fingers. Pout lips in a small circle, as though ready to whistle. Suck in air vigorously through the mouth with sibilance and blow out the cheeks so that they are puffed up. This is called *Kaki mudra* (crow's beak gesture) Now, keeping nostrils tightly closed, create pressure inside mouth as though blowing your nose (as you might do in an airplane to equalize pressure in ears), forcing air into the Eustachian tube. Lower chin to rest on sternal notch. Hold breath as long as possible. Then return neck to upright position, open eyes, exhale slowly through nose, and return cheeks to normal.

This exercises the face muscles, gives cheeks color, strengthens teeth, cures gum and mouth disease, heals skin disease, heals ear problems, prevents deafness, and awakens clairaudience.

Griva-Shakti-Vikasaka
(Strengthening the neck)

Eyes open, relax neck, keep chin in. Rotate and jerk head toward your right shoulder as far as you can, and look toward the right. Then jerk the head toward your left shoulder and look left. Repeat at least 10 times.

Next, jerk head forward to touch the sternal notch and backward to nape of the neck. Repeat at least 10 times.

Then, keeping chin in, try to touch your right shoulder with right ear. Then, try to touch your left shoulder with your left ear. While doing this, don't raise the shoulders. Repeat at least 10 times.

Lastly, keeping chin in, rotate your head in circles, clockwise and counterclockwise, at least five times.

Skandha Tatha Bahu-Mula-Sakti-Vikasaka (Strengthening shoulder blades and joints)

Arms at sides with palms facing inward toward thighs; tuck thumbs into clenched fists. Pout mouth into crow's beak shape. Suck in air and puff out cheeks. Hold breath and lower chin to sternal notch. Keeping back straight and arms stiff, pump shoulders vigorously up and down as many times as possible. Then raise head, open eyes, relax arms, and exhale slowly through nose. This tones the shoulder bones, blood vessels, muscles, and nerves.

Bhuja-Bandha-Sakti-Vikasaka (Strengthening the upper arms)

Arms at sides with palms facing inward toward thighs; tuck thumbs into clenched fists. Bend arms at elbows and raise forearms to a 90 degree angle. Punch fists forward and backward vigorously with a jerk at shoulder level, parallel to ground. Elbows don't go further back than starting position. Repeat 10 times. This develops strong biceps and slenderizes heavy arms.

Kaphoni-Sakti-Vikasaka (Strengthening the elbows)

Arms at sides with palms facing toward front; tuck thumbs into clenched fists. Keeping upper arms rigid and elbows still, raise fists forward with a jerk until they almost touch shoulders. Then jerk them down until they nearly touch thighs. Repeat 10 times. This gives strength and symmetry to forearms, strengthens joints, and improves circulation to arms.

Purna-Bhuja Sakti-Vikasaka
(Developing the arms)

Arms at sides with palms facing inward toward thighs; tuck thumbs into clenched fists. Inhale through nose and hold breath. Keeping arms rigid, swing arms forward from shoulder joints in large circles, as many times as you can. When you can no longer hold your breath, stop, bend arms at elbow, and breathe out forcefully, with a hissing sound, while thrusting fists forward at shoulder level. Then repeat while swinging the arms backward.

Vaksa-Sthala-Sakti-Vikasaka
(Developing the chest)

Arms at sides with open palms facing inward toward thighs. While inhaling through your nose, raise arms and reach hands up as high as you can. Bend backward from waist as far as you can, and look back as far as possible. Hold pose as long as you can while holding breath. Then bend forward while exhaling until you resume erect posture. This pose strengthens chest and back muscles, strengthens lungs and heart, oxygenates blood, and keeps back straight.

Kundalini-Sakti-Vikasaka
(Developing the power of the mystic coil)

Stand erect with feet about two inches apart. Kick your buttocks with your heels, one after the other, in turn. Bring foot back to its original position each time. Repeat 10 times. This exercise awakens *kundalini shakti* (see page 127.)

Jangha-Sakti-Vikasaka
(Developing the thighs)

Keep arms rigid at sides, open palms facing inwards towards thighs. Start doing jumping jacks. Inhale as you jump into the air while you thrust arms straight up. Exhale as you jump back down to original position with arms straight down.

Jangha-Sakti-Vikasaka
(Developing the thighs)

Stand erect, feet together. While inhaling through your nose, do a deep knee bend. Hold arms at shoulder height, parallel to ground, palms down. Stop when thighs are parallel to ground and hold as long as possible. Keep feet flat on ground and knees together. Rise gradually while exhaling.

Pada-Mula-Sakti-Vikasaka
(Strengthening the soles)

Stand up on your toes and then down on your soles. Raise and lower body like this a minimum of ten times. Then jump up and down at least 10 times while balancing only on your toes.

Janu-Sakti-Vikasaka
(Strengthening the knees)

Bend the right leg and touch the buttock with the heel. Then thrust it forward with a jerk at the knee. Do the same with the left leg. Repeat at least five times.

Uddiyana Bandha
(Abdominal lock)

Stand with feet about 24 inches apart. Bend slightly forward at hip and bend knees slightly, until you firmly grasp right thigh with right hand and left thigh with left hand. (See *Figure 8a*.) Blow out forcefully several times to empty the lungs. Then, without inhaling, contract the abdomen forcefully, drawing it upward high into the thoracic cavity. Distend and contract abdomen in rapid succession as many times as possible. Inhale and slowly stand up again. Breathe normally and rest.

Uddiyana Bandha improves breathing and vitality, strengthens abdominal muscles, improves digestion, aids elimination, prevents hernia, aids sexual continence, and awakens kundalini.

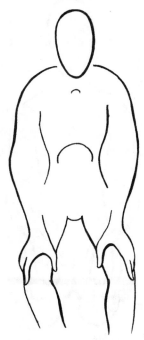

Figure 8a.

Moola Bandha
(Rectal lock)

Stand with feet about 18 inches apart. Exhale completely. Then, while inhaling, make buttocks rigid while forcefully drawing up anal sphincter muscle and genital organs. Hold this bandha as long as possible. Then let go and exhale. Moola bandha stimulates pelvic center, prevents genital, bowel, and bladder diseases, heals frigidity, impotence, hemorrhoids, and prostate.

Yoga Asanas

In this section you'll find traditional Yoga postures. The way to perform these is to assume the described position and then hold the body steady in that pose for a few seconds. Do these to the best of your ability. Stretch only to the point where you feel your muscles stretching; then stop and hold the pose for the time allotted. Keep breathing slowly, through your nose, as you hold the posture (unless otherwise specified). Don't ever push farther than your body wants. Otherwise you might strain or injure yourself.

In addition to the many benefits described for each posture, all the postures have the following benefits: improve circulation, flexibility and posture, lubricate joints, increase longevity and alertness, massage internal organs, stimulate nerves, stretch and strengthen muscles, and promote health and well-being.

Vajrasana
(Kneeling pose)

Kneel down. Sit on heels with spine erect, gazing forward as shown in *Figure 8b/1*. Hold 10 seconds while breathing slowly. Say the following affirmation aloud (or something similar): "Radiant light and energy flow through my being now."

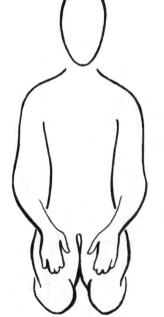

Figure 8b/1.

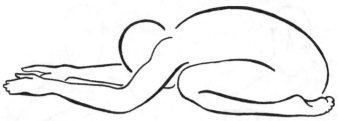

Figure 8b/2.

Take a deep breath. While exhaling, gradually lean forward until forehead touches floor, while still sitting on heels. Stretch out arms in front with palms down. (See *Figure 8b/2.*) Hold five seconds. Then inhale and slowly return to upright position.

Vajrasana can shorten sleep. Practice for five minutes after meals to speed digestion.

Body Tone-up

Stay in Vajrasana (kneeling pose). Massage entire body, step-by-step, by pressing and releasing. Begin by placing hands, palms down, on top of head. Press and release, moving hands down over forehead, eyes, cheeks, front of neck, and chest, as though moving your blood toward the heart. (See *Figure 8c/1* on page 110.) Then, start again at top of head, pressing and releasing gradually, while moving hands over top of skull, back of head, back of neck, around top of shoulders toward the heart.

Place hands on lower abdomen. Squeeze abdomen and move hands upwards, pressing and releasing, proceeding toward the heart. Then begin at back of waist, moving upward. Press and release lower back, upper back, sides, and move gradually toward the heart.

Then squeeze left hand with right hand, pressing and releasing. Move up the inside of fingers, palm, wrist, lower arm, inside of elbow, upper arm, left armpit, left side of chest, toward the heart. Then press and release outside of left fingers, back of left hand, wrist, lower arm, elbow, upper arm, shoulder, and chest. Do the same on right hand and arm, while squeezing and releasing with left hand. (See *Figure 8c/2* on page 110.)

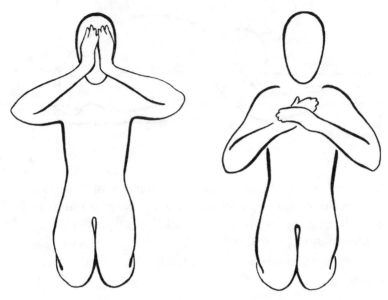

Figure 8c/1.   Figure 8c/2.

Next, unfold legs. Grasp left toes with hands, right hand on the bottom and left on top. Squeeze the toes, pressing and releasing. Then move hands up left foot, ankle, lower leg, knee, thigh, buttock, abdomen, back. Press and release while moving all the way to heart. Do the same with right toes and then press and release gradually, moving toward the heart. *(See figure 8c/3.)*

This tone-up activates acupuncture meridians and increases life energy.

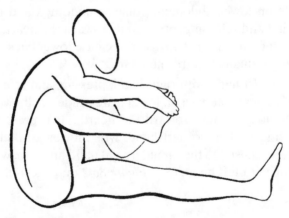

Figure 8c/3.

Suptapavana muktasana
(Lying wind-relieving pose)

Lie on back on asana mat, legs extended. Take a deep breath. Hold breath while bending right leg. Use both hands to put pressure on knee and pull thigh against abdomen as shown in *Figure 8d*. Keep left leg straight. Then exhale while straightening right leg and place it on floor. Now do the same with left leg. Repeat this exercise three times per leg, alternately. Then breathe normally, bend both legs, and press both thighs into abdomen. Clutch knees to chest, lift head slightly, and roll body left and right onto the mat five times per side. Finally, clutch knees to chest, lift head slightly, and rock on spine from neck to tailbone, up and down, five times in each direction.

This posture releases excessive gas, improves digestion, relieves arthritis, and eliminates back pain.

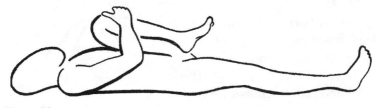

Figure 8d.

Paschimottanasana
(Back-stretching pose)

Remain on back. Place arms above head and stretch entire body, reaching back with fingers and forward with heels. Keeping thighs and legs firmly on floor, gradually curl spine, vertebrae by vertebrae, from neck to tailbone, until you assume a sitting position. Take a deep breath and exhale while bending forward at hip joint, until head touches knees. Grasp big toes with index fingers. (See *Figure 8e* on page 112.) Hold posture five seconds. If it's difficult to touch toes, just bend to the extent you can. Inhale while slowly uncurling spine, vertebrae by vertebrae, and sit back up. Then lie flat on back again.

Paschimottanasana heals skin disease, slims waist, stimulates appetite, eliminates parasites, relieves diabetes, arthritis, sciatica, backache, and leg pain, improves sexual continence, promotes charisma, and generates pleasant body aroma.

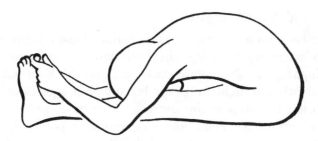

Figure 8e.

Urdhvasarvangasana (Shoulder stand)

Stay flat on back with arms at sides. Raise legs slowly until toes point towards ceiling. Then curl spine upwards gradually, vertebrae by vertebrae, as you support your back with hands while elbows and upper arms rest on floor, until finally your chin presses against chest as shown in *Figure 8f*. Head, neck, and shoulders should touch the mat while doing this asana. If you can't lift trunk all the way up, lift as much as you can. Hold posture 10 seconds while breathing slowly. From this position, go directly into next asana—plow pose.

This pose reduces fat, improves body odors, helps digestion, slims waist, prevents hair graying, improves memory, intellect, concentration, hearing, and eyesight, heals uterus pain, stimulates thyroid and parathyroid, and increases charisma. High or low blood pressure or hernia patients must consult doctor before trying such gravity-inversion postures.

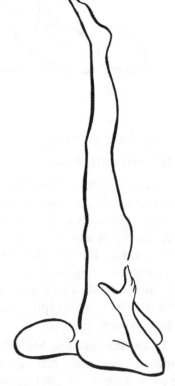

Figure 8f.

Halasana
(Plow pose)

While still in shoulder stand asana, bend at hip joint. Keep legs straight until toes touch the floor behind head. Press chin against chest. Place arms and hands in front of you with palms flat on floor as shown in *Figure 8g*. If you can't touch toes to floor, just go as far as you can. Hold position ten seconds. Then bend knees and gradually uncurl spine, vertebrae by vertebrae, from neck to tailbone, while supporting back with hands, until buttocks return all the way to floor. Then straighten legs and lower them slowly. Do this asana slowly and gracefully, without rushing. Don't shake or jerk your body.

Halasana (also called *Sarvangasana:* all-limb posture) improves eyesight, stimulates thyroid and parathyroid, eliminates skin disease and menstrual pain, improves body odors, reduces fat, and prevents senility. Heart disease or high blood pressure patients must not try this.

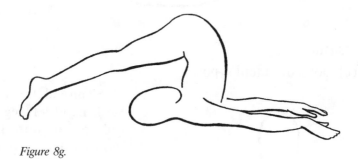

Figure 8g.

Ustrasana
(Camel pose)

Lie on mat, face down. Bend knees and lift up legs while firmly grasping right ankle with right hand and left ankle with left hand. While breathing in, raise head, neck, chest, and knees by tugging on ankles. Arch spine until whole body forms a bow. Rest entire body on abdomen. (See *Figure 8h* on page 114.) Relax and maintain posture five seconds, while holding breath. Then exhale and breathe normally, release ankles, and slowly come out of pose. Lie flat on mat on stomach.

Ustrasana (also known as *Dhanurasana*: bow pose) heals rheumatism, diabetes, constipation, and stomach disorders, aids digestion and appetite, reduces fat, and relieves female disorders. Hernia patients must avoid this asana.

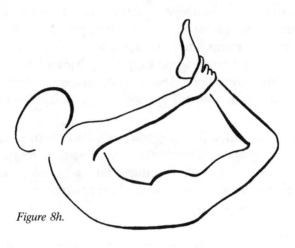

Figure 8h.

Siddhasana
(Perfect pose or adept's pose)

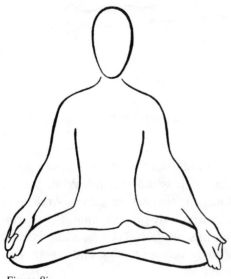

Figure 8i.

Sit up and stretch legs forward. Bend left leg at knee and place left heel at perineum, the soft portion between anus and genitals. Then bend right knee and place right heel against pubic bone, just above genitals. Arrange genitals so no pressure is felt. Place toes of both feet between thighs and calves. Keep spine straight and place hands on lap, palms up, right hand over left. Or as shown in *Figure 8i*, place hands on knees, palms up, touching tips of thumbs to tips of index fingers allowing other fingers to relax (to ground the body). Close eyes and say the following affirmation aloud, "I AM a perfected being of great power and energy" (or similar). Hold posture ten seconds and breathe normally.

Siddhasana is rated foremost of all 840,000 asanas. The best asana for meditation, concentration, prayer, self-realization, and worship, it helps attainment of *siddhis* (perfections or supernormal powers), promotes *Brahmacharya* (celibacy) and mental discipline, raises *prana* (energy in the breath) through the *nadis* (subtle nerves) and awakens *kundalini* ("serpent power" or subtle energy in the spine).

Padmasana
(Lotus pose or foot lock)

Sit on mat and stretch legs forward. Grasp right foot and place right foot over left leg onto left thigh, near hip. Then grasp left foot and place over right leg onto right thigh, near hip, with heels touching each other as close to navel as possible. (See *Figure 8j.*) Keep head, neck, and trunk erect. Place hands between heels, right over left, with palms up. Or place hands on knees, palms up, touching tips of thumbs to tips of index fingers, allowing other fingers to relax. Keep both left and right knees and thighs flat on floor. If you have difficulty getting into lotus pose, then do "half-lotus," placing right heel against perineum and left foot on right thigh. Hold lotus posture ten seconds while breathing normally.

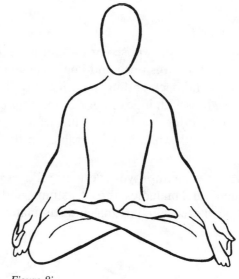

Figure 8j.

Lotus pose improves digestion, breathing, concentration, steadiness, and calmness, relieves constipation, indigestion, and flatulence, and benefits female organs.

Yoga Mudra
(Lotus pose with forward bending)

Stay in lotus pose (or half-lotus). Inhale deeply and then exhale while bending forward until forehead touches floor as shown in *Figure 8k*. Be sure to bend at hip joint rather than just waist. Stretch arms out in front with palms down. Hold posture five seconds. Then inhale while uncurling spine slowly, until you're once again sitting straight in lotus pose.

Yoga Mudra relieves abdominal disorders and improves digestion.

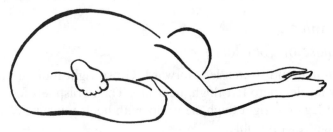

Figure 8k.

Matsyasana
(Fish pose)

Remain in lotus pose (or half-lotus). Then bend backwards, keeping feet locked in lotus pose and knees remaining on floor. Place elbows on mat and bend back and neck until top of head rests on floor. If you can, grasp big toes with index fingers. *(See Figure 8l.)* Hold asana five seconds. After completing asana, slowly uncurl neck, flatten back, and then gradually raise trunk while keeping palms on floor. Once again you're in lotus pose.

Matsyasana improves eyesight, relieves constipation, diabetes, uterus and menstrual maladies, throat, asthma, and bronchial disorders, moisturizes skin, increases charisma, and stimulates thyroid and parathyroid.

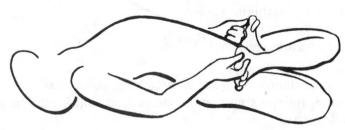

Figure 8l.

Bhujangasana
(Cobra pose)

Turn over on mat and lie on stomach with face down. Position hands just below shoulders with palms down. While inhaling, slowly lift head and bend spine, vertebrae by vertebrae. Keep hips and legs on floor. Don't jerk while raising torso, but bend gracefully and slowly. Mostly use back muscles rather than arms to raise the body. When you reach your point of maximum bending, look up as far as you can as shown in *Figure 8m*. Remain in position five seconds while holding breath. Then exhale while uncurling spine, vertebrae by vertebrae, until you're once again lying flat on the floor. Repeat.

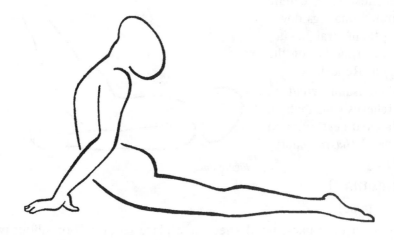

Figure 8m.

Bhujangasana relieves constipation and indigestion, broadens chest, slims waist, relieves back pain, strengthens abdomen and eyes, increases body heat, and heals menstrual ailments, ovaries and uterus. Hernia patients must not perform this asana.

Salabhasana
(Locust pose)

Remain on mat, lying on stomach. Place hands parallel to body at sides, palms up. Rest chin on mat and clench fists. Inhale slowly while you stiffen body, point toes, and raise legs and sacrum high off ground, without bending knees. Keep thighs, legs, and feet in straight line. Lift legs to your greatest extent, without straining. (See *Figure 8n.*) Remain in posture five seconds. Then exhale and slowly bring legs down, keeping them straight, until you are lying flat on the mat again. Repeat.

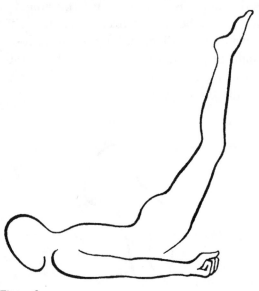

Salabhasana broadens chest, relieves constipation, stimulates digestion, and opens navel *chakra* (energy center).

Figure 8n.

Chakrasana 1
(Wheel pose)

Roll over onto back, bend knees, and place feet on floor, about two feet apart from each other, near buttocks. Then bend arms, lift elbows, and place palms on floor just behind shoulders. Lift body into arched position. Bend spine as much as possible by walking hands towards feet. (See *Figure 8o* on page 119.) Breathing normally, hold pose five seconds, or as long as you can. Then slowly bend arms, bring torso down, bend knees, and lie on back again. Rest for a few seconds.

Chakrasana broadens chest and slims waist.

Paschimottanasana
(Back-stretching pose)

Sit up. Repeat head-knee pose (on pages 111 and 112) and hold for five seconds. Then sit up slowly.

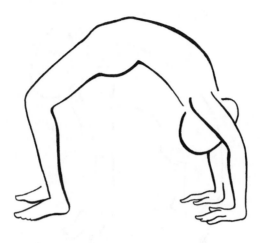

Figure 80.

Chakrasana 2
(Wheel pose)

Kneel down in Vajrasana (kneeling pose). Raise upper legs until thighs are perpendicular to lower legs. With knees a few inches apart, bend spine slowly, vertebrae by vertebrae, until you grasp left ankle with left hand and right ankle with left. (See *Figure 8p* on page 120.) If you have difficulty grasping ankles, just bend back spine as far as you can, without straining. Inhale deeply and hold breath while remaining in posture five seconds. Then exhale, let go of ankles, raise spine, vertebrae by vertebrae, and slowly bend neck and head forward. Then sit back down into Vajrasana (kneeling pose).

This asana (sometimes called *Ustrasana:* camel pose) broadens chest and slims waist.

Mayurasana
(Peacock pose)

Stay in Vajrasana (kneeling pose). Then place knees about 18 inches apart, lift thighs, and bend forward while placing palms on mat, about two

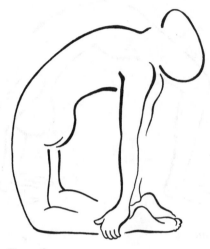

Figure 8p.

inches apart, fingers facing backwards or sideways, depending on which is more comfortable. Place upper arms against chest with elbows together, pressing into navel. Inhale while leaning upper arms and elbows into chest and abdomen until forearms and hands support the entire torso. Place forehead on floor. Slowly straighten legs, point toes, and allow toes to rest on floor. Lift head and look forward. Then slowly lift legs until head and toes are level with each other, parallel to floor. (See *Figure 8q* on page 120.) If you have difficulty raising legs, keep toes on mat until you gradually build strength. Hold posture five seconds. Then rest toes on mat and exhale.

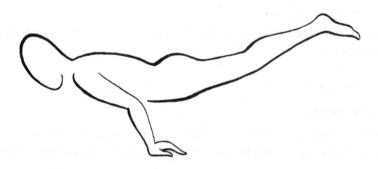

Figure 8q.

Gradually come down from pose and rest on the mat for a few minutes. (Don't attempt this asana without medical permission.)

Mayurasana relieves abdominal disorders, improves digestion, heals liver and spleen, improves eyesight, increases breathing, improves balance, and awakens *kundalini shakti.*

Ardha Matsyendrasana
(Half spinal twist)

Come out of Vajrasana and sit on floor with knees bent. Place right foot under left buttock with heel at perineum. Then bend left leg and place left foot to the outside of right knee, as shown in *Figure 8r.* Then twist spine slowly, vertebrae by vertebrae, twist neck, and look toward left as far as you can. Twist right shoulder until right arm is placed on left side of left leg. Grasp left foot firmly with right hand. If you can't grasp left foot, just reach as far as you can, without straining. Then curve left arm around back and reach for right hip. Hold pose five seconds. Then release hands, slowly untwist spine, vertebrae by vertebrae, and unbend legs. Repeat the same posture, twisting towards right.

Ardha Matsyendrasana rotates vertebrae, awakens *kun-dalini,* stimulates gastric secretion, eliminates intestinal parasites, heals diabetes, rheumatism, and disorders of liver, spleen, and gastrointestinal tract, and strengthens eyes.

Padahastasana
(Hands to feet pose)

Stand up. Inhale deeply, bend neck and look up as far as you can while raising arms over head with upper arms touching ears. Then slowly bend forward at hip joint while exhaling, until fingers touch toes and head touches knees as seen in *Figure 8s.* Keep ears in

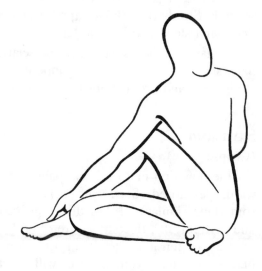

Figure 8r.

contact with arms while bending forward. Then place palms on floor and
bury head between knees. If you can't complete posture, bend as far as
you can without straining. Be sure you bend
mostly at hip joint and rather than just waist.
Stay in posture five seconds. Inhale while
slowly raising body, uncurling vertebrae by vertebrae, until you're standing again.

Padahastasana broadens chest, slims
waist, reduces weight, increases height,
lengthens muscles, reduces abdominal fat, and
develops graceful figure.

Konasana
(Angle pose)

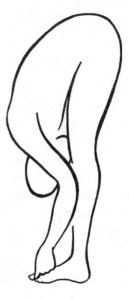

Figure 8s.

Remain standing and place feet far apart,
as shown in illustration. Lift arms to shoulder
height, palms down, while inhaling slowly. Exhale while gradually bending to left until left
hand touches left ankle. Stretch right arm toward left, resting it on right side of head, as
shown in *Figure 8t*. If you're unable to touch
ankle, bend as far as you can without straining. Remain in posture five
seconds. Slowly rise back to upright position. Repeat on right side. Practice asana slowly, without jerking.

Konasana relieves backache and sciatica, relieves lung ailments, eliminates skin disorders, invigorates appetite, aids elimination, increases height,
straightens and proportions body. Can be practiced by pregnant women

Savasana
(Corpse pose)

Lie down on mat on back, palms up, legs relaxed, toes pointed outward, eyes closed. (See *Figure 8u*.) Say the following affirmation aloud (or
something similar), "I AM divine peace and harmony." Breathe slowly
and rhythmically. Become aware of body. Anywhere you feel a sensation
of stress or tension, allow your attention to quietly rest on that place or
places. Gradually your muscles will relax and become soft and pliable.

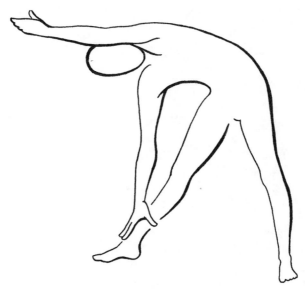

Figure 8t.

Your mind will settle down. Your spirit will become tranquil and content. Stay in this pose at least five minutes.

Savasana relaxes body, increases blood flow, oxygenates blood, eliminates toxins, reduces tiredness, improves alertness, eases mind, raises spirit, and prepares body for deep meditation and spiritual awakening.

> *"Do not neglect this body. This is the house of God; take care of it. Only in this body can God be realized."*
> —Nisargadatta

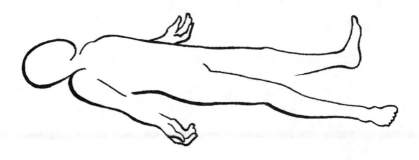

Figure 8u.

Chapter 9

reater Power Through

Yogic Breathing

In This Chapter:
- Discovering Prana Power.
- Awakening Kundalini and Chakras.
- Practicing Pranayama.

Chapter Affirmation:
"I AM perfect balance and equilibrium."

Have you ever noticed breathing is irregular, broken and heavy when you're under stress, yet it's regular, smooth, and slow when you're at peace? Breath is the key to inner peace and tranquillity.

Breath alters, depending on how vital or dull, robust or sickly you feel. Babies breathe naturally, with vigor. Children's breathing is rapid, keeping pace with a small body in continual motion. Teenagers stop their breath due to awkwardness. Adults, habituated to breathing breathlessly, curtail breathing. The elderly fight for each breath with effort.

The life force or vital energy in breath is called *prana* in Sanskrit and *chi* in Chinese. Hatha Yoga uses breathing exercises, *pranayama,* to awaken prana. In fact, the word *hatha, ha* (sun) and *tha* (moon), means solar and lunar breaths, which are *prana vayu:* positive vital air, and *apana vayu:*

negative vital air. Regulating and harmonizing prana brings steadiness of mind. Conversely, stilling the mind through meditation harmonizes and regulates the breath.

Prana is universal energy that gives life to matter, the power within everything, animate and inanimate. It's in the air, but isn't oxygen or any other physical constituent of air. It's in every particle of creation, but isn't a particle. Prana is entirely non-material.

The Power of Prana

The dormant spiritual force within everyone can be awakened by using prana consciously. Thought is the most refined, potent form of prana. The movement of the lungs is the weakest. Filling the body with pranic energy can bring healing and vitality to every cell.

Pranic energy can be transferred. Anyone coming into proximity with a prana-filled person receives this energy by osmosis. The most powerful speakers, biggest celebrities, greatest politicians, revered prophets, successful businessmen, captivating movie stars, alluring women—all owe their fame to abundant pranic energy. Magnetic personalities have a knack for influencing others by their speech, even their mere presence.

Spiritual masters, overflowing with prana, transmit pranic energy to heal and uplift people, even bring them to higher consciousness. Prana is key to the secret of divine transmission from *guru* (teacher) to *chela* (student).

By practicing pranayama (Yogic breathing methods), you can collect and conserve pranic energy in your solar plexus, the pranic storage battery. Prana power can increase your charisma, will, influence, and supernormal powers to such a degree that you can sway the world.

Everyone uses pranic energy. When you need to lift a heavy object, solve a complex problem, or overcome danger, what's the first thing you do? Your first impulse is to hold your breath. This draws on an extra supply of pranic energy to accomplish the task.

You can use prana for healing, as long as you know how to replenish it from the infinite source. Have you ever stroked a sick friend's forehead? In that loving act, you transmit prana to him or her. When you're injured, first you unconsciously hold your breath, then touch your body. Your instincts know about prana, even if your conscious mind doesn't.

By practicing pranayama, you can tap the vast power within the breath and use it for self-healing, to heal others, even the entire planet.

Conserving the Power in Breath

Yogis believe that when you're born, your life span is predetermined. Your length of life is counted by your number of breaths, not by your number of years. This is one reason Yogis are concerned with conservation of prana.

Pranic energy is continually drained by every thought, word, and deed, and then replenished by every breath. Other sources of prana are sunlight, water, air, and food. Prana is absorbed by skin from fresh air and daily bathing, by the tongue through prolonged chewing, by nostrils and lungs.

Moderate exercise, such as walking, bicycling, swimming, and asanas, along with proper breathing and pranayama, oxygenates blood and revitalizes vital energy—without the strain or oxygen debt of heavy exercise.

When you inhale, prana enters your body and gets stored in your nerve centers, particularly the solar plexus. The more prana you receive, the more vital you become. Proper breathing can prevent disease and increase will power, concentration, self-control, and spiritual awakening.

Deep meditation automatically controls breathing, which becomes slow, regular, and quiet. In the state of *samadhi* (equanimity of mind and body), your breath becomes so refined that it's imperceptible. You seem to hold your breath altogether. In fact, your breath isn't being held, it's being held in suspension, neither breathing nor not breathing.

If this sounds scary to you, it isn't. You won't pass out by practicing meditation. You won't die from samadhi—just the opposite, in fact. You'll become more alive, awake, and healthy.

How can meditation cause your breath to settle down to near nothingness? As mental activity becomes subtle and quiet, physical activity relaxes and metabolic functions decrease. Energy is conserved. Heart rate slows. Breath rate lessens until it attains suspension. The mind and body become quiet and silent, like a still pond without a ripple. Such is samadhi, the experience of Yoga.

Awakening Kundalini Shakti

Your physical body is just one of your many bodies. You have a subtle nervous system with an entire complex of *nadis* (nerve tubes) and *chakras* (nerve plexuses) running through it. Prana, in the form of nerve currents, travels through ten of the nadis, energizing the body.

Of the 72,000 nadis, the one most vital to pranic energy is *kundalini shakti* (serpent power or mystic coil). Normally kundalini is asleep, coiled near the tail bone at *brahmarandhra mukha* (mukha means mouth), the base of the nerve tube *sushumna nadi,* which runs through the spinal cord into the brain, until it reaches *brahmarandhra,* a nerve complex at the top and middle of the head, about five fingers back from the hairline. Sushumna is usually closed at the lower end, with no prana passing through it.

Two nadis (nerves), *ida* and *pingala,* wrap around the sushumna like a caduceus. They correspond to the left and right sympathetic cords in the body, which control afferent (sensory, which carries sensations to the central nervous system) and efferent (motor, which carries commands to the body) nerve currents.

Prana normally flows through ida and pingala. Pranayama can force prana to withdraw from ida and pingala, open sushumna nadi, flow into it, and travel up the spine. The rising kundalini awakens supernormal powers. When it reaches *brahmarandhra* at *sahasrara chakra* (thousand-petaled lotus), Yoga (divine union) is achieved and limits of time, space, and causation are transcended.

Some ways to awaken kundalini shakti are devotion, worship, meditation, will power, discernment, knowledge, and body purification. Any manifestation of spiritual gifts or supernormal powers indicates kundalini is awakened to some degree.

Kundalini shakti is personified as the Divine Mother: Shakti Ma, Kali Ma, or other female deities. She's the feminine power at the base of the spine, which unites with the masculine power in the brain, her consort, Lord Shiva. The divine union of Shiva with Shakti in the sahasrara chakra is likened to a sexual coupling or a marriage. This union of opposites is a powerful symbol depicted in all cultures (see *Figure 9a*).

Divine Union of Opposites

Female	Male
Darkness	Light
Yin	Yang
Moon	Sun
Receptive	Projective
Passive	Active
Subjective	Objective
Yoni	Linga
Holy Spirit	Father God
Shekinah	YHVH
Shakti	Shiva
Prakriti	Purusha
Anima	Animus

Figure 9a.

Opening the Chakras

Students have repeatedly asked me to write about *chakras*. Therefore, in this book I've included simple ways to begin to awaken kundalini shakti, including meditative practices, physical exercises, and pranayama. Yet, I wouldn't recommend more advanced practices without the benefit of a spiritual master. This section is a brief introduction to the chakra system.

The word *chakra* means wheel in Sanskrit. Chakras are circular centers of subtle energy that appear like lotus flowers. They correspond to the nerve plexuses and organs in the physical nervous system.

Kundalini shakti traveling up the spine in sushumna awakens the chakras. It is believed that kundalini vibrates with the sounds of the Sanskrit alphabet, which is built by this internal experience of the chakras. Every letter of the alphabet is contained in, and important to, the chakra system. The specific Sanskrit letters appear on the lotus flower petals on each of the seven chakras and give rise to the form of a presiding deity. For a visual representation of each of the seven chakras listed here please refer to *Figure 9b.*

1. *Muladhara*, at the base of spine and sacral plexus, associated with organs of excretion, represents *prithivi tattwa* (earth element) and sense of smell. The mantra of this chakra is *lam:* लं. Its form is a four-petaled lotus and a triangle with kundalini shakti in the center. The Sanskrit letters on its petals are semivowels: *vam:* वं and sibilants: *sham, shham, sam:* शं, षं, सं. Brahma, the Creator, is its deity. This center is the seat of primal life energy.

2. *Swadhisthana,* in the genitals and prostatic plexus, associated with gonads, represents *apas tattwa* (water element) and sense of taste. *Vam* is its mantra: वं. Its form is a circular moon with a six-petaled lotus. Its letters are labials: *bam, bham, mam:* बं, भं, मं, and semivowels: *yam, ram, lam:* यं, रं, लं. Vishnu is the presiding deity. A bright crescent moon is in its center. This center is the seat of creativity.

3. *Manipura*, at the navel and solar plexus, associated with pancreas and abdominal organs, represents *agni tattwa* (fire element) and sense of sight. The form is triangular, the mantra is *ram:* रं and deity is Rudra. It has ten petals. Its letters are cerebrals: *dam, dham, nam:* डं, ढं, णं, dentals: *tam, tham, dam,*

Chakras

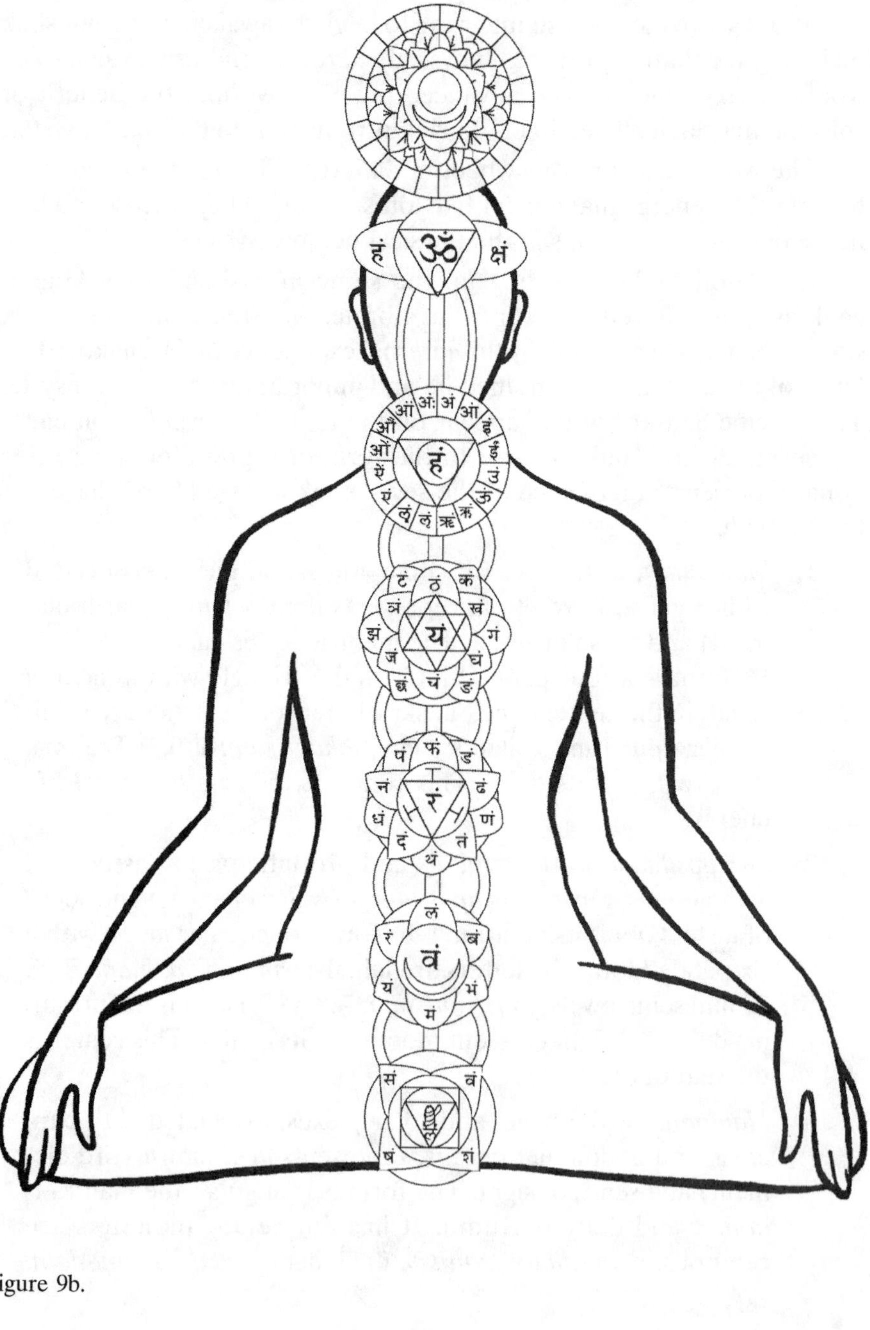

Figure 9b.

cerebrals: *dam, dham, nam:* ड, ढं, णं, dentals: *tam, tham, dam, dham, nam:* तं, थं, दं, धं, नं, and labials: *pam, pham:* पं, फं. This center is the seat of will, ego, feelings, and subconscious emotions.

4. *Anahata,* at the heart and cardiac plexus, associated with thymus and lungs, represents *vayu tattwa* (air element) and sense of touch. Its mantra is *yam:* यं, deity is Isa and form is a six-pointed star with twelve petals. Its letters are gutturals: *kam, kham, gam, gham, nam:* कं, खं, गं, घं, ङं, palatals: *cham, chham, jam, jham, nam:* चं, छं, जं, झं, ञं, and cerebrals: *tam, tham:* टं, ठं. This center is the seat of love.

5. *Vishudha,* at the throat and laryngeal plexus, associated with thyroid, represents *akasha tattwa* (ether element). The mantra is *ham:* हं, deity is Sada Shiva, and form is a triangle with 16 petals. Its letters are vowels: *a, aa, e, ee, u, uu, kr, kree, lre, lree, ye, yai, o, ow, aam, ah:* अं, आं, इं, ईं, उं, ऊं, ऋं, ऋं, लृं, लृं, एं, ऐं, ओं, औं, आं, आ:. This center is the seat of creative expression and communication.

6. *Ajna,* between the eyebrows, corresponding to cavernous plexus, associated with pituitary gland, is the "third eye" of higher mind, clairvoyance, knowledge, divine experiences, intuition, spiritual discernment, and higher voice. Ajna is the seat of *sukshma prakriti* (primordial power of everything) and *atman* (soul). Its form is a triangle with two petals with letters *ham* and *ksham:* हं, क्षं. Its mantra is *aum:* ॐ and deity is Paramashiva (Shambu).

7. *Sahasrara,* in the brain, associated with pineal gland, is *brahmarandhra,* thousand-petaled lotus. When kundalini first reaches sahasrara, it remains only momentarily and then returns to Muladhara. Only by consistent practice does divine union become permanent. When Shakti unites with Shiva in this center, the perfected *siddha* becomes *jivan mukti* (liberated soul), dwelling in eternal bliss, possessing all powers.

The Five Pranas

Prana, the life force in breath, takes five separate forms in your body. The five pranas work through the nerve plexuses in the sympathetic part of the autonomic system to receive or generate *vayus:* nerve currents or impulses. Each prana is governed by a vayu. These five vital airs *(pancha prana)* or vital forces, breathe life into your body:

1. *Prana* is inward and downward motion. Seated in the heart, it works through the cervical (throat) plexus, governing speech, voice, respiration, and movements of the gullet. Prana vayu is generated by inhaling.

2. *Apana* is downward and outward motion. Seated in the anus, it governs excretion, kidney, bladder, genitals, colon, and rectum. It works through the lumbar (mid-back) plexus. Apana vayu is generated by exhaling.

3. *Samana* is horizontal motion. Seated in the navel, it regulates digestion, stomach, liver, pancreas, and intestine through the thoracic (chest) sympathetic autonomic system.

4. *Udana* is upward and outward motion. Seated in the throat above the larynx, it regulates swallowing, falling asleep, and controls all automatic functions in the head. At the time of death it separates the astral body from the physical body.

5. *Vyana* is circular motion. All-pervading and moving through-out the body, it controls circulation of blood, directs voluntary and involuntary movements of muscles, joints, tendons, and fascia, and keeps the body upright through unconscious spinal cord reflexes.

During the practice of pranayama (Yogic breathing), *prana vayu* is gen-erated by inhaling, and *apana vayu* by exhaling. Prana vayu is an afferent impulse (going to the brain) and apana vayu is an efferent impulse (mov-ing from the brain and nerve centers). While the breath is held, the two vayus unite in *Muladhara* (sacral chakra), generating tremendous prana to awaken kundalini lying dormant at the base of the spine.

Suppressing natural body urges cuts off the natural flow of prana, which causes imbalance and disease. Thirteen urges that allow natural flow of prana are to:

1. Defecate.	5. Belch.	9. Drink.
2. Pass gas.	6. Yawn.	10. Cry.
3. Urinate.	7. Vomit.	11. Sleep.
4. Sneeze.	8. Eat.	12. Pant after exertion.
		13. Ejaculate.

Secrets of Breath

Yogic breathing is complete breathing. What does that mean? Your chest and abdomen are separated by your diaphragm. As you inhale, the ribs move outward and the diaphragm contracts and moves downward. This movement expands the lungs. Hence, the diaphragm is the key to absorbing the most pranic energy during breathing.

To demonstrate this, let's try an experiment:

1. Sit up straight. Take in a big deep breath while moving the diaphragm downwards. Don't raise your chest or shoulders. If you're doing this right, your belly will distend as you inhale.

2. This time take a big deep breath while expanding the chest, but don't let your diaphragm move or allow your belly to distend.

3. Now as you take a big deep breath, don't let the diaphragm move, and at the same time, raise your shoulders.

Now try these three styles of breathing again until you determine which style takes in the most air. The first way of breathing, called "deep breathing," "low breathing," or "diaphragmatic breathing," brings significantly more air into the lungs. The second, "chest breathing," brings less. The third, "high breathing," the worst, causes many respiratory diseases, such as asthma.

Now try another experiment:

Sit up straight. Put your left hand on your belly and right hand on your upper chest. Take three deep breaths. Notice whether your belly distends as you inhale (as it should) or contracts (as it shouldn't) and whether your shoulders rise while breathing (as they shouldn't). Do you take shallow or deep breaths?

Although diaphragmatic breathing is the best of the three styles of breathing, it still isn't complete breathing. During low breathing, the lower and middle parts of the lungs expand. In chest breathing, the middle and part of the upper lungs expand. In high breathing, only the upper part expands. However, In Yogic breathing, the lungs expand entirely.

Ordinary exhalation releases just a small pocket of air from the upper part of the lungs. But Yoga breathing releases a maximum quantity of stagnant air from the lungs to allow more prana to enter. That's why, during pranayama, the number of seconds for exhalation and inhalation is counted, usually at a ratio of two to one.

Beginner's Breathing Exercise

Let's learn our first breathing exercise now. It's a simple method to get into some new breathing habits. By the way, the best time to do breathing exercises is right after asanas and before meditation.

Sit up straight. Put left hand on belly and right hand on upper chest. Take five deep breaths. Make sure, as you inhale, first your belly expands, then chest expands, then upper chest expands, using deep, chest, and high breathing. As you exhale, belly and chest contracts. Don't raise the shoulders at any time.

Now repeat exercise, only this time, count the seconds as you breathe. Count three seconds as you inhale and six seconds as you exhale. Take five deep breaths like this. Do this exercise for a week.

During second week, take 10 deep breaths and increase the number of seconds to four for inhalation and eight for exhalation. During third week, take 15 deep breaths and practice five seconds to inhale and 10 to exhale. During fourth week, six seconds to inhale and 12 to exhale.

By doing this exercise, you'll learn to breathe properly, expand lung capacity, and begin to purify the nadis (nerves). Once you've practiced this exercise for a month, discontinue it and begin the next exercise: Yogic alternate breathing.

Alternate Breathing Exercise

Do you notice at any given moment one of your nostrils is more open and the other more blocked? You'll recognize this if you sleep on your side, since you can breathe better through one nostril.

But did you notice that clear breathing automatically switches from one nostril to the other from time to time? If you're in excellent health, this alternation takes place regularly, approximately every hour and 50 minutes.

Your right nostril's breath, connected to pingala nadi, is believed to be hot. So its breath is called "sun breath," which generates body heat, raises metabolism, and accelerates the organs. The left nostril's breath, said to be cool, is "moon breath," connected to ida nadi. Its energy cools the body, lowers metabolism, and inhibits the organs.

If the breath flows through one nostril more than two hours, the body is unbalanced—too much heat or cold. If ida is overactive, mental activity wanes and lethargy increases. If pingala is overactive, then nervous activity rises and mental disturbances result. If breath flows through one nostril for 24 hours, it's a warning of illness. The longer breath continues in one nostril, the more serious the illness will be.

Yogic alternate breathing, *Anuloma Viloma Pranayama,* equalizes the sun and moon breaths. By breathing through one nostril, then the other, you'll create equilibrium in body metabolism and purify the nadis.

Let's do it now!

Anuloma Viloma Pranayama

Sit up straight. Close right nostril with right thumb. Exhale completely through left nosril for 12 seconds, contracting belly and chest. Inhale noiselessly and completely through same left nostril, expanding belly and chest, for six seconds. Then immediately close left nostril with middle and ring fingers of right hand. Now exhale for 12 seconds, fully and noiselessly, through right nostril, contracting belly and chest. Without stopping, close right nostril again with right thumb and repeat process. Do this 15 to 20 times.

Once you've mastered six seconds to inhale and 12 to exhale, gradually increase to seven and 14 seconds, then eight and 16. Do this only after practicing several months.

By practicing this pranayama, your breath becomes regular and deep, health improves, body gets lighter, and eyes shine. These changes indicate the nadis are purifying. Health benefits include stress reduction, calmness, slower heart rate, and lower blood pressure.

Having mastered the alternate breathing pranayama, you can practice a more advanced version after a few months:

Do the same alternate breathing exercise, but add retention of breath. Inhale (pooraka) for four seconds, hold breath (kumbhaka) 16 seconds, and exhale (rechaka) eight seconds. After one month, increase ratio to five seconds to inhale, 20 to retain, and ten to exhale. Gradually increase until you attain eight, 32, and 16 seconds.

"No one is free who is not master of himself."
—William Shakespeare

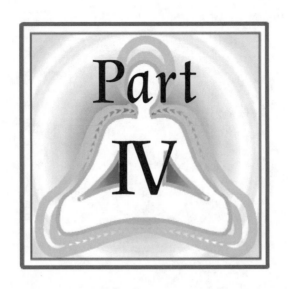

Part IV

Discovering Karma and Past Lives

Chapter 10

ispelling Myths

About Karma

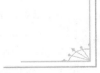

In This Chapter:
- Taking Personal Responsibility.
- The Law of Karma.
- The Law of Grace.

Chapter Affirmation:
"I claim my good, very good, perfection now."

You can view your life in one of two ways: Either you're in charge, and life is in your hands; or you're a passive observer, and life is "done to" you. If you subscribe to the first way of thinking, then you're a master of destiny. If you believe the second, then you're a victim. To which category do you belong, and where do you want to belong?

You have an inner divine power that isn't influenced by external circumstances. With that power at your command, you can do anything. Anything means *anything*. You aren't subject to environmental conditions. By tapping into divine power and using it, you can rise above these conditions. But the power requires some effort and practice to master.

Self-mastery means achieving your dreams, attaining happiness, and fulfilling your heart's desires. You can take command of your life. In this section of the book, you'll learn how.

Determinism: Fact or Fiction?

Does some outside force control you? Is your fate determined by a punishing, condemning God, or by chance, luck, or accident? In truth, there are no accidents. You aren't prey to winds of fate. Everything that happens "to you" is caused by your thoughts, speech, and actions, not by anything or anyone else.

Today a sickness, perpetuated by fatalistic psychics, astrologers, and fortune-tellers, runs rampant. This illness of "determinism" presumes your destiny is already written.

Often you hear, "You can't change the stars," "I guess it was meant to be," "It must be for the best," "Maybe I wasn't supposed to get it." Is some unseen force controlling you? Are you a victim, a passive audience watching a play, or are you in the starring role? I contend that you're not only the actor, but also the playwright. You've written the script yourself.

No mysterious force is plotting your future. You might believe external forces shape your life, such as environment, social status, race, sex, family, upbringing, or education. But these were all chosen by you.

At each moment you have nearly limitless choices. Before birth you decided what you wanted to accomplish and then chose the parents and family most conducive to your desires and life path. Yes, you did read that right. Believe it or not, you chose your own parents before you were ever born!

At every step you make decisions. Based on these choices, you make new ones. All your choices are determined by free will. It's useless to praise or blame others for fortunes or misfortunes that happen "to you."

Barbara Gianino, one of my students, says: "I used to blame my unhappiness on how I was raised, my parents, the job situation, or other situations in life outside of myself. Now, I recognize I am responsible for what I experience. I draw to myself these things because of my belief system. And if I don't like something, I recognize that I can change this. I now know how to ask for any error-belief in my subconscious mind to be healed and that the truth replace that." (More about this in the next chapter.)

What Is Karma?

Do you struggle to get what you want? How can you fulfill desires and manifest your dreams? The answer is hidden in the "law of _karma._" Sir

Isaac Newton said: "Every action has an equal and opposite reaction." Jesus stated: "Whatsoever a man soweth, that shall he also reap."[1] *Karmic* law means action-and-reaction or cause-and-effect.

Many people believe that whatever you do will be done back to you. In other words, if you kill someone, then later in this life or a future life, someone will kill you. Does this happen? Surprisingly, the answer is no.

Karma is a Sanskrit word that simply means "action." That's all it means. It doesn't mean good deeds are rewarded while bad deeds are punished. There are no karmic debts from past lives to punish you in future lives. Nor do karmic courts or trials judge, sentence, or execute you in retribution, ad infinitum.

How does the law of karma actually work? Whatever you do, think, or say produces far-reaching consequences. When you drop a pebble into a small pond, ripples radiate outward in concentric circles. When these circles reach their outer limit, they begin an inward journey, creating new ripples converging towards the center. In the same way, even your imperceptible thoughts affect the universe more profoundly than you could imagine.

Along similar lines, Jesus said, "As ye would that men should do to you, do ye also to them likewise."[2] Every moment you radiate either harmonious waves of thought energy, or inharmonious waves. Positive feelings create an *aura* (vibrational field) that attracts good by the law of magnetic attraction (like attracts like). Happiness or suffering is the result of whatever you project into the universe.

The karmic law can be used to your advantage, for "as thou hast believed, so be it done unto thee."[3] This means whatever you believe will happen is exactly what will happen. Your deepest convictions influence what you think, say, and do, which, in turn, determine your destiny.

If you believe you deserve punishment due to past "evil" deeds, then you'll be punished, for "it is done unto you as you believe." If, on the other hand, you think God is all-loving and doesn't demand retribution, then you won't be punished. If you believe losing weight is difficult, then it will be. If you believe you're poor, you will be. If you believe you're lonely, you will be. If you believe you're happy, you will be.

"It is done unto you as you believe" means that *you're* in charge, not a karmic judge sitting in the sky recording your deeds in a big book, conjuring punishments to deliver in your next incarnation. You aren't a marionette, and God isn't a puppeteer.

Your Subconscious Tyrant

Which beliefs are implied in the statement, "It is done unto you as you believe"? Conscious or subconscious? First let's define "conscious" and "subconscious." Right now you're conscious of reading this book, of sitting on a chair, of sounds, sights, and smells. That's your conscious, waking mind, otherwise known as "attention."

In contrast, your subconscious mind is an impartial computer bank that indelibly records every experience. For instance, in childhood, if a teacher said, "You're a brilliant student," that statement left an impression. If your father said, "You're a bumbling idiot," that negative statement also left its impression. As a teenager perhaps you were spurned by your true love, and you felt devastated and undesirable.

Memories gestate in your subconscious mind and become a set of conditioned beliefs or patterns. Your every decision is based on beliefs stored in that subconscious computer bank.

Here's an example: Gerald wants to own a Jaguar. So he cuts out a picture of a Jaguar from a motor magazine and pastes it on his refrigerator, because he attended a seminar about how pictures fulfill desires. Next he repeats affirmations: "My Jaguar is coming," "I have a Jaguar now." He asks someone to pray for his Jaguar, and he waits for the Jaguar to fall out of the sky and plop onto his driveway.

But, a deep unconscious belief hides in Gerald's mind. His deepest conviction is that he *deserves* a Hyundai. What does Gerald get? That's right, he gets the Hyundai, because his subconscious belief determines the outcome.

In this case, Gerald's subconscious mind is his master, and his conscious mind is its slave. His hidden beliefs have dominion over him. As long as Gerald continues to fall under this subconscious spell, he'll get into situations that he hasn't sought or requested intentionally.

Can Gerald get out of this predicament?

In anthother instance, one of my students named Charlotte Mitchell was a bookstore owner in Toronto. She had bought expensive subliminal tapes to lose weight. But she gained 20 pounds listening to the tapes! Why? Because her subconscious mind denied every affirmation. Her mind won each internal battle and evidently won the war. Reprogramming the subconscious mind may not be as easy as you think.

Can anyone escape subconscious tyranny?

Your Ego Box

Your ego is an amalgamation of beliefs that you've come to accept and own. A psychological term, called "identification," indicates a small ego box that defines you. This limited identity, within small boundaries, determines your choices and therefore your fate.

But who are you in *reality*? Indeed, this question is elementary. You've already read the answer in previous chapters of this book: "I AM love, I AM light, I AM a child of God, I AM divine Spirit."

But do you really know this, or are you kidding yourself? Is it just an intellectual exercise to speak the words, "I AM divine"? Most people, when confronted with this dilemma, admit their incapacity to know, on the deepest level, who they really are.

Identifying yourself as the limitless divine self can only be known by direct experience in a higher state of awareness—not in ordinary waking state. During deep meditation you can know by direct revelation, "I AM divine, I AM perfection everywhere now, I AM that I AM."

Such a revelation releases previously held beliefs. Your old identity ego box gets traded in for a new one, a box without sides, top or bottom, infinitely large, flexible, and unbounded. This new identity defines you as Spirit, your true nature.

Your new level of consciousness brings peace, comfort, and divine direction. Then you operate from divine will rather than ego will. No longer do you identify with frustration and failure. No longer is it impossible to manifest your dreams. Now you have support from the creator of this universe, the one omnipotent power that brings spontaneous fulfillment of desires.

Lord Shankara (509-477 B.C.), a great Hindu saint, said, "Cease to identify yourself with race, clan, name, form and walk of life. These belong to the body, the garment of decay. Cease to follow the way of the world, cease to follow the way of the flesh, cease to follow the way of tradition. Get rid of this false identification and know the true Atman [higher Self]."

Your Internal Judge and Jury

Humanity's beliefs are stored in an aggregate collective mind: thoughts of reward, punishment, condemnation, retribution, and conditional love. From an early age, were you taught if you were good, you'd be rewarded, and if you were bad, you'd be punished? Are you still operating under a need to be approved as a "good" child?

This belief in "good and bad"/ "right and wrong" is so ingrained that we don't think twice about it. Authority figures, such as parents, teachers, churches, and the media, brainwashed us with societal rules and judgments. Now that we're grown, our inner jury (subconscious mind) follows the same rules, doling out rewards and punishments based on "good" or "bad" behavior.

Tens of thousands of thoughts go through your mind every day. If these thoughts condemn you, then the result is inevitable. Do you punish yourself with self-destructive experiences? *Even at this instant*, are you feeling guilty about your past self-punishments? Amazing how the mind works, isn't it?

Your subconscious computer continually compares your current behavior with idealistic past models. If your inner jury deems it "good," then a prize is awarded by your inner judge. If it's "bad," then a punishment is imposed by your inner sheriff. Then the law of karma, which fulfills every subconscious request, delivers it.

Here's an example: Maggie's husband criticized her early in the morning and she felt guilty and unworthy. She became impatient during breakfast and yelled at her children, because she felt unloved and blamed her husband. After the children left for school, Maggie felt even worse because she yelled and wasn't more patient. She wasn't a "good" girl.

Then Maggie set out for the grocery store. She didn't see a car coming from the left at an intersection. This car hit hers and she was injured as a result. Voilà: Maggie's punishment! Her thoughts of guilt projected into the universe. She subconsciously demanded punishment. Her karmic parcel arrived in the form of an automobile accident.

Every situation is a result of subconscious demands made by each person involved. Others fulfill your needs, and you fulfill others' needs, even if those needs don't make a whole lot of sense. The need to be victimized seems fairly irrational. Yet its cause is that person's unconscious guilt and desire for punishment.

Karmic deliveries may come immediately or perhaps in a future incarnation. That's why infants or young children suffer. Or why some people lead charmed lives.

Karmic results come individually or collectively. Groups of people demand collective punishment and thereby cause natural disasters, plagues, or wars. Every subconscious demand for reward or punishment is fulfilled by the impartial law of cause and effect.

The karmic law may be a hard pill to swallow. It's difficult to accept that the poor, the afflicted, disabled, ill, maimed, homeless, even babies and small children—all unconsciously magnetized devastating experiences by their own subconscious need to be punished.

The good news is the relentless karmic law can be used to magnetize good. It isn't necessary to punish yourself anymore. You're the sole author of your destiny, so write a new, better life. Since self-judgment caused your problems, you can forgive yourself and reverse this downward spiral. Control your subconscious mind rather than letting it control you.

Your Divine Wish-Fulfilling Tree

Do you believe Spirit wants to fulfill your desires? Or is God vengeful, demanding, and capricious? You were probably taught that God punishes or rewards you depending on whether you're "good" or "bad."

Contrary to popular belief, God isn't keeping track of your actions. Only you are. God doesn't "reward" or "punish" you, depending on how "good" or "bad" you are. Only you do. God doesn't place demands or conditions and can't be bribed by "good" or "bad" deeds. God doesn't respond to bribes. God is, in fact, completely unconditional and un-bribable.

God is doing one thing only: fulfilling your desires. In fact, you receive exactly what you place on your order form. God is an infinite shipping department whose only mission is to fill your orders. Your every thought is a prayer, a request to satisfy a desire. God, in infinite mercy, impartially and unconditionally fills every subconscious request.

A popular concept today is that we're in "earth school," to learn lessons. Do you believe a divine schoolmaster dispenses tests, lessons, and trials? If you believe you must learn "lessons" through "trials," then that's exactly what you'll get. If you believe you don't need trials or suffering, then you won't need these in order to "grow." "It is done unto you as you believe."

For example, Stacey was speeding on the highway and got into a terrible car accident. She had to stay in the hospital for six weeks. After Stacey's recovery, she said philosophically, "Oh, it was 'good' that I had an accident; I learned a 'lesson' that I should be cautious and slow down when I drive."

Was it "good" to have an accident? Is it necessary to be hospitalized in order to "learn" to drive slowly? If you create a "mental law" of punishment, lessons, and trials, that's precisely what will happen. Your life can be a glorious celebration of ease, joy, harmony, love, abundance, and fulfillment. Just heal your mental law and let Spirit give you good.

Your Mental Legislature

Often students ask me, "What about the hardened criminal who has no remorse? According to your theory, he'll get off scot-free. Where's his punishment?"

Let's consider this criminal's subconscious mind, filled with negative thoughts. You may think he's without remorse because of his tough façade, but his subconscious mind believes in self-punishment as much as anyone else. His hate, anger, fear, resentment, and cold-heartedness inevitably attract violent, negative experiences. Whether or not the court inflicts punishment, he'll punish himself for his crime by the law of magnetic attraction, which attracts like to like, either in this lifetime or a future life.

Your entire set of beliefs, called your "mental law," is determined by past experiences, upbringing, and societal influences. Whatever rules you buy into become your mental statutes. Each new experience adds more statutes. You operate under an intricate set of rules. But, since you have freedom of choice, you can obey your self-imposed mental law, or you can disobey its rules and make new ones.

Under what mental law do you operate? What subconscious statutes govern your life? No genius is required to figure this out. Simply look at your life as it is right now.

Now let's do an exercise. Pretend you have an empty slate on which to write your destiny. On the left side, write a set of laws you'd like to be governed by. On the right side, write the laws you've been governed by so far. Your slate may look something like this:

Laws I Would Like	Laws I Have Experienced
1. I always get what I want.	1. I rarely get what I want.
2. I always have all the money I need.	2. I never have enough money
3. I am a very happy person.	3. I am not very happy.
4. I have a lot of friends.	4. I have very few friends.
5. I love my work.	5. I hate my work.
6. I have a harmonious family.	6. I have a difficult family.
7. I feel easy in social situations.	7. I am socially uncomfortable.
8. I am slim and trim.	8. I can't lose weight.
9. I have perfect eyesight.	9. I can't see without glasses.
10. I have a wonderful love relationship.	10. I have no love in my life.

This exercise will help you get in touch with the statutes of your personal mental law. The beliefs you've accepted as absolute truth, your deepest convictions, will determine your destiny.

You're the creator and maintainer of limiting laws that give rise to a restricted pathway. You can also break the shackles of those limitations. You are, in reality, perfect and unlimited. So create a mental law for yourself of good, good, and very good!

Three Types of Karma

Please refer to the chart "Karma" on page 148. The sum total of memories and experiences from all your past lives is called *sanchita karma* in Sanskrit. That's your big mountain of karma. When you incarnate, you break a chunk off the mountain. This chunk, *prarabdha karma,* is based on your choices, beliefs, thoughts, and habits. Prarabdha karma determines your experiences in this lifetime and helps you accomplish your goals.

Free will, *agami karma,* conceives of creative solutions to karmic situations. Those choices are implemented by *kriyamani karma:* thoughts, words, and deeds created each moment. Free will can mitigate future events. However every decision is largely based on past experiences.

Here's an example: Phil was raised in a poor family, had a low-paying job, and considered himself a second-class citizen. His boss invited him to a party at an opulent mansion. A beautiful woman arrived in an expensive car, unescorted. She slunk out of her car and breezed by Phil, smiling with welcomeness. He was taken by her beauty and felt she was attracted to him. But a nagging voice inside said, I'm undeserving. Even though he wanted to ask her to dance, he didn't. Paralyzed by shyness, Phil missed the opportunity and went home depressed and lonely. He created kriyamani karma corresponding to his prarabdha karma, his past beliefs about himself.

However, Phil could take charge of his destiny and conceive of a better solution. He could use agami karma to transform his unworthiness into self-confidence and then use kriyamani karma to make different decisions. Phil could create new karma: a wonderful new relationship with an attractive woman.

Your prarabdha karma is of three types: *droodha, adroodha,* or *droodha- adroodha.* These measure the severity of your belief pattern.

Karma

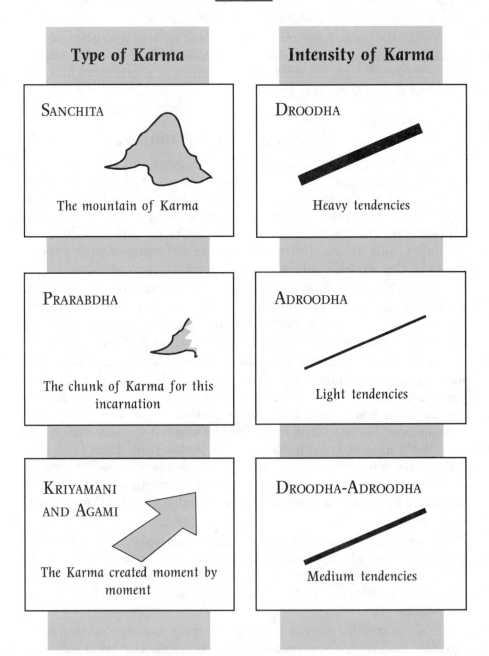

Type of Karma	Intensity of Karma
SANCHITA — The mountain of Karma	DROODHA — Heavy tendencies
PRARABDHA — The chunk of Karma for this incarnation	ADROODHA — Light tendencies
KRIYAMANI AND AGAMI — The Karma created moment by moment	DROODHA-ADROODHA — Medium tendencies

Figure 10a.

1. Droodha is defined as difficult to overcome, like a line etched into stone.

2. Adroodha is easy to overcome, like a line drawn in the sand.

3. Droodha-adroodha is in between, like a line etched on a piece of wood.

For instance, suppose that maintaining loving relationships is easy for you. Imagine, however, that it's impossible to make money. Then, in the area of money, you would have negative droodha karma. Each person's karma is different. Some find it easy to manipulate certain areas of life that others find difficult.

It's difficult to fulfill what you know is difficult to fulfill. It's easy to fulfill what you believe you can fulfill. Simple, but true. I've never met a person who prays for things they can get without effort. They only pray for things that are difficult to get.

Do the Stars Rule You?

Do you believe your fate is determined by the stars? Well, it isn't. Your astrology chart doesn't determine your destiny. *You* do. You picked your moment of birth based on your plan for this incarnation. A definite pattern, represented by the placement of planets in our solar system, existed when you took your first breath. These planetary positions are a blueprint, a map of your beliefs (your mental law).

Some astrologers are capable of reading this map accurately. They can foresee the exact timing of events based on this blueprint. But they're not reading planetary influences. They're reading your own beliefs and choices. Your astrology chart shows exactly what will happen if you continue to foster the same beliefs you had at birth.

Your soul precisely calculated your birth time and place, where the stars were aligned in a configuration that perfectly reflected your choices at the time. However, your choices and beliefs can change any moment. So you have complete control over your astrology chart. It doesn't control you. Your mental law, which you had at birth, can be transformed into a new set of laws and a new destiny. You are in charge.

How Grace Overcomes Karma

Because of God's benevolence, a "law of grace" can reverse and overcome any and all mental laws. The law of grace states: "With God, all things are possible."[4]

The law of grace nullifies the mental law of karma. Grace operates under divine rules, not limited by human beliefs and conditions. This divine law functions when you lift your consciousness to a higher level, into direct contact with Spirit. "But if ye be led of the Spirit, ye are not under the law [the law of karma]."[5]

The more you connect with Spirit, follow inner divine guidance, and surrender your ego to divine will, the more grace becomes potent in your life. In harmony with your true purpose, your desires attune to divine desires. Your mind is one with divine mind. Your heart beats with the heart of God. Your body becomes an instrument for God's symphony to play. Your breath is the breath of the almighty. Your life is divine life.

Jesus and other masters demonstrated the law of grace operating continually in their lives. With this divine law, miracles occurred, incredible healings took place, even the dead were resurrected.

The law of grace instantaneously dispels all limiting beliefs. If you believe you're subject to karmic law, then you will be, for "it is done unto you as you believe." Once you accept the law of grace, then the spell of karma is broken and no longer controls you. You're free from all past "sin." "For sin shall not have dominion over you: for ye are not under law [law of karma], but under grace."[6] And, "As the blazing fire turns fuel to ashes, O Arjuna, so does the fire of wisdom turn all actions (karma) into ashes."[7]

When a diseased woman touched the hem of Jesus' garment, he said, "Thy faith hath made thee whole."[8] At that moment the law of grace overcame her mental law which caused her illness for 12 years. Through faith she was healed instantaneously.

The law of grace works through faith. Faith is the healer, the miraclemaker, the power that says, "All things are possible."[9] Faith can heal the statutes of your mental law and allow you to consciously write your own laws of destiny.

Faith is the key that unlocks the door to the immutable law of grace, the law of bountiful mercy that forgives all "sin" (error thinking) and all "debts" (belief in reward and punishment). God, the all-forgiving, grants unlimited pardon for "wrongdoings," and, in unconditional love, bestows divine grace, the tangible, earthly proof of God's existence and God's love.

What Are Your Choices?

Life is simple. You have two basic choices each moment: be happy, or suffer. You may argue that you don't have control over whether you're happy or you suffer. However, if you're not in control, then who is?

You may believe societal influences are in control. If so, then why does one sibling suffer and another experience happiness? You may think God is in control. The notion that someone somewhere in the sky arbitrarily decides which of your actions are punishable, remembers these actions, and then imposes verdicts, is absurd.

You have freedom of choice and are fully responsible for everything that happens. Get over the idea that you're a victim. Your life is simple. You can walk the path of happiness and love, or suffering and fear. You create heaven or hell by your choices. Choose the light or the darkness. You're in charge, so choose well.

> *"He that makes his bed ill, lies there."*
> —George Herbert

Chapter 11

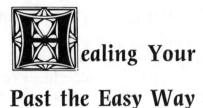

ealing Your

Past the Easy Way

In This Chapter:

- The Power of Affirmative Prayer.
- Healing Your Present Life.
- Healing Past Lives.

Chapter Affirmation:

"I AM the healing power of God."

The most troublesome thing about the law of karma is that your present choices are based on past experiences. Therefore you're bound by the past, to the degree you buy into it. Most people say you can't change the past—or can you? Is it possible to transform past impressions, conditioning, and negative emotions? Can you heal blockages preventing you from making wise choices? From this moment on, can you write your life on a clean slate?

Your *sanskaras* (past memories, seeds of desire) are held in your *chitta* (subconscious mind). That's your storehouse of impressions, your computer hard drive that holds all memories. Whenever you need to make a decision, your mind searches that database to draw on similar experiences. If your database consists of fear, doubt, timidity, and confusion, you won't make the wisest choices.

The good news is you have free will and power to heal your past. You can change your mind at any time. By realizing what needs healing, and then using the power of your word in prayer, you can heal anything. In this chapter, you'll learn some ways to do that.

The Power of Your Word

Let's do an experiment. First drink a glass of water. Then sit comfortably and take a few deep breaths. Now place your middle finger over your index finger, resting the tip of your middle finger on your index finger's fingernail. Got it? Good. Now, say the following words, out loud, in a strong, clear voice. "I AM a mighty, powerful, spiritual being." Now try to push down on the fingernail of your index finger with the tip of your middle finger.

This time, once again rest the middle finger on the index finger. Now say, aloud, "I AM a miserable sinner." Now try to push your index finger down again.

Once again, rest the middle finger on the index finger. Now say out loud, "I AM divinely protected by the light of my being." Once again, try to push your index finger down with your middle finger.

What did you discover? Did you notice the muscles in your index finger weakened when you spoke negatively and strengthened when you spoke positively? You've just demonstrated the power of your word through a method called "muscle testing."

Every thought, word, and deed has power—power to strengthen and bring happiness, or power to weaken and cause suffering. You may not easily have control over every one of your thoughts, but you can definitely control your speech. Therefore, be careful about what you say, because speech produces inevitable results.

By using the words "I AM," you invoke the mighty "I AM" presence, your powerful "I AM" self. Whenever you invoke the "I AM," be sure that whatever you place after those words is something you want to own. By saying, "I AM sick," "I AM poor," "I AM depressed," you will surely manifest these results. Use the "I AM" wisely with such words as, "I AM happy," "I AM content," "I AM healthy." Your words have more effect than you can imagine, so use them carefully.

For instance, the words, "I'll never get a good job," reverberate throughout the universe. By repeatedly affirming this, you won't get a good job. If you continually affirm, "I always have all the money I need," those words will cause you to have the money you need.

You've just learned how to use the power of your word for good—to heal, transform, and achieve your goals. Verbal affirmations and prayers are specific statements, spoken aloud, that can effect powerful healing. Now you're going to learn some specific affirmations to help you do that.

Let's get started!

Are You a Psychic Sponge?

One of my students from New York said to me, "I get so drained. I feel exhausted all the time. I'm like a psychic sponge. People around me are psychic vampires, draining my energy, sucking me dry. I feel like a wet mop that's been dragged through the mud all day. By the end of the day, I'm so tired that I can't do anything. I just flop onto my bed, utterly exhausted."

Does this sound familiar? If so, then you're a psychic sponge. That means you absorb vibrations like a sponge absorbs water. Empathy indicates that you're intuitive. But it's counter-productive to be overly sensitive or to let others control and diminish you so much that you no longer exist.

Here's a self-authority affirmation for all you empaths. In fact, it's for everyone, to help you maintain inner integrity:

> "I AM in control. I AM the only authority in my life. I AM divinely protected by the light of my being. Thank you God, and SO IT IS."

Say this affirmation out loud in a strong, clear voice whenever you feel intimidated, drained, overly sensitive, afraid, or out of control. Use it before meditation and before sleep. If you're a healer, psychic, or therapist, then say it before and after each client. Use it before any important meeting, especially with an authority figure. It's powerful, and it works.

What Imprisons You?

A psychic tie is an undo attachment or repulsion to anything that has control over you: a person, place, thing, organization, situation, circumstance, memory, experience, or addiction. Psychic ties can be seen clairvoyantly as ropes, cords, strings, bonds, or ties. Often they're attached to your energy centers, like umbilical cords. Nearly everyone has psychic ties, and no one needs them.

Many people mistake psychic ties for love ties. True love bonds are unbreakable golden ties that maintain loving relationships. Psychic ties, on the other hand, are chains of attachment and psychic imprisonment.

What causes a psychic tie? It's residue from an argument or another emotional encounter. It's the need for a substance that rips at your soul. It's whatever tugs at your mind. It's obsession, addiction, or co-dependency.

Let's learn how to cut psychic ties using a simple affirmation. Read it aloud in a strong clear voice. In the blank space, say the first person or thing that comes to mind:

"I now cut any and all psychic ties between myself and _____ (*person, place, thing, etc.*)____. These psychic ties are now lovingly cut, lifted, loved, healed, released and let go by the divine presence. Thank you God, and SO IT IS."

If you cut psychic ties daily with the people with whom you live and work, I guarantee you'll have more loving, more intimate relationships with those people. Do it. It works!

Are You Plagued by Negative Emotions?

Negative thoughts and emotions trouble just about everyone. No matter how depressed, worried, angry, confused, or hopeless you feel, you can heal yourself and others through the power of prayer. Here's how: First, figure out what you're feeling. That's essential, since nothing can be healed without knowing what needs healing. Second, use a simple formula to heal it. Sound easy? It is. Let's do it now.

1. Get comfortable, close your eyes, and take a few deep breaths. Now get in touch with whatever negative thoughts or emotions are coming up for you. Maybe you feel fear, doubt, limitation, confusion, anger, unworthiness, lack, guilt, worry, or sadness.

2. Now open eyes and write a list of your emotions down the left side of a sheet of paper. Then, next to each item, write their opposite counterparts. For example, if you wrote "hate," write "love" next to it. If you wrote "confusion," write "clarity." If you wrote "doubt," write "certainty," and so forth.

3. Now read the following affirmation out loud in a clear voice. In the first blank space, say all the negative emotions listed on the left side of your paper. In the second blank space, say their positive counterparts:

"I invoke the divine presence to help me eliminate negations and limitations that prevent me from knowing the truth of my being. I now dispel all negations of ___ *(list negative emotions you want to release here)* ___ and all other thoughts and emotions that do not reflect divine light. Instead, I now welcome feelings of ___ *(list positive emotions you want to accept here)* ___. I AM now in control. I thank God, AND SO IT IS."

This thought-form healing affirmation seems so simple that you might doubt it would work. But it does work—every time. It's amazingly powerful. This simple prayer can heal *anything*—any mental, physical, emotional, or spiritual problem.

Now that you know this prayer, you no longer have an excuse to stay in a bad mood. Let's put it this way: You can mope around as long as you want. You can feel bad if that makes you feel better. But if you'd rather take responsibility for your bad mood and change it, just get out this book and read the healing prayer.

Do You Have Unwanted Invaders?

Have you ever heard of the astral world? It's a level parallel to this earth plane, but in another dimension, inhabited by souls who didn't enter the divine light after death.

Perhaps you've read about the near-death experience, in which a person flatlines (brain activity and breathing stops) for a few minutes and then revives. Many near-deathers have a common experience: They see a tunnel, a road, or a bridge ending in a brilliant light. By entering that light, they meet a divine being or deity. Then a panoramic life review begins—a rerun of life, like a movie, not only from their perspective, but also from the viewpoint of everyone else they ever encountered.

I'm convinced this is exactly what happens after death. But some deceased souls don't enter that light. Why? A few reasons are: unfinished business, attachment to loved ones, loved ones holding them back, attachment to materialism, addictions to substances, fear of hell, guilt or feeling undeserving, disbelief in the afterlife or in God, stubbornness, arrogance, confusion, mistaken beliefs, ignorance of their death. As a result, such souls become earthbound spirits, discarnate entities.

Because they no longer inhabit a body, certain lost souls may be so driven to continue earthly existence that they take possession of a live body. Any susceptible human is fair game. What makes you prey? Debilitating influences, such as: addictions to drugs, alcohol, sex, or food, or a sudden accident or illness. If you're weak, an earthbound entity can attach itself to you. Then, under astral influence you might exhibit strange new behavior or sudden personality changes, such as drug abuse, which the possessing entity indulges in through your body.

How to prevent astral possession or influence? Keep your aura closed off by using the following affirmation:

"I AM in control. I AM the only authority in my life. I close off my aura and body of light to all but my own divine self. Thank you God, and SO IT IS."

Astral entities are usually lost, confused souls trying to find their way home. Their motives can be harmless and playful, or mischievous and malevolent. But, whatever their motives, they can be healed and sent to the divine light by using a simple astral healing formula. Say this out loud in a clear voice:

"Beloved ones, you are unified with the truth of your being. You are lifted in divine love. You are forgiven of all guilt and shame. You are healed, loosed, and released from loss, pain, confusion and fear. Divine love and divine light fill and surround you now. Attachment to the earth no longer binds you. You are free to go into the divine light now, dear ones. Go now in peace and love."

This powerful prayer can be used anytime you get a yucky, creepy feeling. Yes, you read that right. Yucky, icky, creepy, gooky feelings can be healed with the astral healing prayer. Haven't you ever visited a house with that feeling? Or a hospital, mental institution, bar, prison, school, cemetery, or courtroom? Whenever you're creeped-out, afraid, have a nightmare, or a strange experience happens, use the astral healing prayer. This prayer is never wasted. Even though most souls go into divine light after death, there are still so many lost souls that one is always within earshot.

What about Past Lives?

Why would you want to remember past lives? Some people are curious about the past. Was I famous, rich, beautiful? My question would be: "Why jump into a trash bin and wallow in garbage?" If there's a purpose for digging out the garbage, fine. Otherwise, let the sanitary engineers haul it away.

Is there a reason to delve into past lives? I can think of some excellent reasons. But they aren't the usual ones. The only time I dig into past lives is to heal something from the present life—something important.

What's important in your life that needs healing? Perhaps you have a phobia, like fear of elevators or planes. Maybe you have a confusing, or even devastating, relationship. Perchance you consider yourself unworthy. Or you're gripped by an addiction. These are all good reasons to heal your past.

Let's learn a simple way to heal deep impressions from past lives, or from your childhood, right now:

1. Decide on a problem you want to heal. Choose only one, for example: fear of intimacy, or fear of fire, or healing a wounded relationship.

2. Sit down and get comfortable. Close eyes and take a few deep breaths.

3. Now get in touch with the problem. That means visualize it, feel it, hear it, taste it, remember it, relive it. Do whatever it takes to get into that state of terror, anxiety, or other emotion. For instance, if you're afraid to fly, remember being on a plane and feel the flood of emotions. To heal a relationship, remember a devastating incident. Continue to imagine your problem until you reach an intensely emotional state.

4. Once you're in an intense state of emotion, then say aloud, "Higher self, please show me the first time that I experienced this feeling in the past."

5. Now take a deep breath; do nothing, nothing, and less than nothing. As you sit quietly, a picture will pop into your mind. Or a smell, or feeling. Or you'll hear something. Then say out loud, "Higher self, please show or tell me where I am." You'll notice your past life surroundings. Then say, "Show me more." You'll remember a past incident related to your current problem. Continue to ask questions until the whole movie plays out in your mind. Then ask your higher self, "Is that all, or is there more to know?"

6. Once you've remembered your past life pattern, you've done 90 percent of the healing. Now do the other ten percent. Say the following affirmation:

"Thank you, Spirit, for showing me this past pattern. I now heal and release all limiting ideas under which I have been operating as a result of past experiences. I accept that I AM healed of the past. I know now that I no longer need to repeat this pattern in this life. Therefore I AM free of this pattern now and forevermore. Thank you God, and SO IT IS."

When to Heal

These healing formulas are powerful tools that you can read more about in my book, *Divine Revelation*. You can use them whenever you or others need spiritual healing. Use them before meditation, before sleep, before going outside, in a crowded place, before meeting someone important. Anytime you're disconnected from divine Spirit, reconnect using these prayers. During meditation, if you're embroiled in negative thoughts and can't go deep, use the healing affirmations. Prayer is a powerful way to stay connected to Spirit.

"If the doors of perception were cleansed, everything would appear to man as it is, infinite."
—William Blake

Chapter 12

aking Your Dreams

Come True

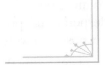

In This Chapter:
- Daring to Dream.
- Getting What You Want.
- Spiritual Mind Treatment.

Chapter Affirmation:
"Every moment is a miracle."

Why were you placed on this earth? You were not tossed onto this planet arbitrarily. You have a divine purpose and destiny that's calling you right now. Everyone is a mighty, powerful, spiritual being.

You've heard this before. Perhaps you read spiritual books about your unlimited potential and great power. Yet you might not be in touch with it. Often our own greatness eludes us. We belittle ourselves and elevate others. But you're no less than, nor greater than, anyone else.

Everyone on earth is a divine being of great power. You were given a divine gift—free will—and can use that gift to uplift yourself and others. You can make a difference on this earth, and you're here for a purpose.

Dare To Dream

As a child you probably imagined how you would contribute to the world when you grew up. Perhaps you saw yourself in a particular profession or field of endeavor. Maybe you dreamt of traveling to foreign lands, or being an artist, dancer, actor, or writer. Maybe you have imagined serving in politics, religion, or charity. Or you wanted your own family and children. Maybe your dream was more abstract, like "world peace," "enlightenment," "God-realization," or "planetary healing."

Whatever your dream was, it may have been shattered by grief or scattered in the wind by necessities of fate. Your beloved dream may have vanished, and with it, all hope and optimism. Your spirit may have died young, along with your dream. Perhaps you continue sleepwalking in "quiet desperation," pretending it doesn't matter. But your true vision, to live the purpose you were born to fulfill, still burns in your heart.

That flame of hope is the divine call to wake up to who you truly are—a powerful, magnificent being of infinite love, light, and power. There's nothing too big or too great to accomplish. You are unlimited. You don't have to give up your dream, no matter what your seeming restrictions or chronological age. With faith and perseverance, you can manifest it. You were born to fulfill your destiny.

Now let's take a test with no grade or studying. Get out a paper and pen and answer one question:

> Imagine for a moment that you have unlimited resources: all the money, intelligence, people, assistance, time, and freedom you could ever need. You have everything at your command, you know everything, you can do anything, no one will criticize you, and you cannot fail. There are no limits. Let your imagination soar to realms far beyond what you normally conceive.

> What would you do in that situation?

Please, don't write about things you would buy. Instead, write what you would do with your days. If nothing comes to mind, just imagine yourself on your deathbed. What would you regret not having done?

Once you've written your paper, read it over and add anything you may have missed. *Do not* read the next paragraph until you've written your paper.

An Amazing Secret

Here's an amazing secret: This paper can completely transform your life. What you've written is your most heartfelt dream, your true desires and higher purpose. You've gotten in touch with your unlimited self and graduated to unbounded thinking.

It might not seem possible to fulfill your dream. You may feel undeserving or restricted. But you *can* start fulfilling it right now, today. Furthermore, you already have the resources to fulfill it. Because it comes from your heart, it's within your grasp. Even if you think you don't have the means today, if you would take just one step in the direction of fulfilling your dream, Spirit would begin to support you.

That one step may involve getting more education or traveling to a different area. It may mean letting go of something holding you back. You may need to give up a dead-end relationship. By taking that first step, you might be criticized as a "dreamer." Your family or friends might laugh.

You may be paralyzed by a plethora of excuses. But you have the power to do it. There's nothing stopping you except yourself. Let go of the idea of not being ready, of not having enough or being enough. Free yourself from the incessant wheel of procrastination.

Nearly everyone who takes a risk is afraid at first. You can be afraid and start anyway. Do you want to fulfill other people's dreams or your own? Set your priorities and live your life with a sense of urgency.

Start on your dream today. Take the first step to fulfill your higher purpose. It takes courage to take that step, but it's definitely worth taking. Ask Spirit to help you.

You can create miracles and fulfill your destiny, whatever it may be. No matter how impossible it may seem now, you can do it. Dare to do it.

In this chapter, you'll be given some tools to help you fulfill your dreams and create miracles. However, your success in using these tools is entirely dependent on your desire to succeed and your willingness to practice. Like any other skill, such as swimming or violin playing, not only knowledge is required, but also practice. You can learn the theory of swimming from a book, but you can't actually swim until you get into the water. The knowledge in a book is dead until you give it life by getting into the pool and swimming.

Getting What You Want, Despite Yourself

It's a good idea to recognize your true desires, because if you don't fulfill them consciously, they'll be fulfilled anyway, much to your inconvenience. Perhaps you don't perceive your deep desire to make a major life change. You may resist that change, even if you intuitively know it's for the best. Desperately you cling to past limitations. What happens? Your mind unconsciously causes so much upheaval that you're forced to change anyway.

For example, Ralph always wanted to become a doctor, but, because he got married early, he never went to medical school. In order to attend school now, he would have to uproot his entire family and move to another city under great financial pressure. So Ralph kept his job as a bank manager in a small town. But deep within, his desire to become a doctor was brewing, sabotaging his life. Unconsciously he caused problems at work and got fired. When, to his dismay, he couldn't get another job, he borrowed money to meet his mortgage payments. His car was repossessed. At the point of desperation, Ralph saw a notice on the Internet about a medical school offering scholarships for qualified applicants. He applied and, lo and behold, he was accepted. Now he had to borrow more money. Under tremendous economic strain he moved his family to a new city to attend medical school. After moving, Ralph said, "It was meant to be. It was all for my good."

What was "meant to be" and "for good"? Certainly the outcome, going to medical school, was good. But was the misery that got him there "good"? If Ralph had made a deliberate effort to attend medical school in the first place, then his move would have been significantly easier. He could have mastered circumstances rather than letting circumstances master him.

You can make positive life changes consciously, rather than unconsciously, by, first, becoming aware of your true desires, and, second, by praying to fulfill those desires.

Are You Praying Backwards?

Bea Wilkinson, an author from Springfield, Missouri, is an expert at practicing prayer and manifesting her goals. Her prayers brought about a wide range of miracles, from healing her husband's cancer to acquiring various Cadillacs. One day she wrote down three wishes: 1. She wanted to visit Mount Shasta, because she heard about its spiritual qualities. 2. She always wanted to experience a Native American sweat lodge. 3. She wanted to go camping, and although she repeatedly told her husband she wanted to go, he never gave her that opportunity.

Later that day, Bea received a phone call from a friend. She was stunned when her friend invited her to a special sweat lodge. It would take place in California, on Mount Shasta, of all places. But, more amazingly, her friend said, "The only glitch is, I'm sorry, but we'll have to camp on the mountain." Bea was thrilled about her trip, to say the least.

The sweat lodge had been built for 25 people. However, Bea was squished into this hellishly hot, miserable, constricted space, mano à mano, with 79 others. Even worse, when she finally escaped from the inferno, she trekked a long distance to a stream to cool off. By the time she arrived, although no longer hot, she jumped in anyway. It turned out to be an icy, glacier-fed stream. Bea rushed back in gratitude to the hellish sweat lodge.

Later that night Bea tucked herself into her tent. But, unknown to her, the air mattress had a hole in it. Needless to say, Bea didn't go camping again. Nor did she ever visit another sweat lodge.

This story has a moral: Be careful what you ask for. You might get it!

The trouble with prayer and manifestation is often people pray backwards. They pray for anything and everything without concerning themselves about the consequences of fulfilling their prayers.

My recommendation is to first discover what is highest wisdom to do, according to your true purpose and heart's desires. Then, when you fulfill your prayers, you'll be in alignment with Spirit. Your goals will manifest more easily when you ask Spirit to advise you first. Be led by Spirit and then pray forwards rather than backwards.

Spiritual Mind Treatment

Spiritual Mind Treatment, otherwise known as Scientific Prayer, is a process of "treating" (healing and spiritualizing) your mind so it can know the truth of divine eternal good behind the appearance of false limitations. Once your mind has been "treated," then it is ready to accept the action of the Spiritual Law to demonstrate (manifest) your prayer. Spiritual Mind Treatment has created miracles in millions of people's lives. Divine Science, Science of Mind, Religious Science, Unity Church, and other "New Thought" teachings all use Scientific Prayer in one form or another.

The New Thought movement is a non-sectarian metaphysical philosophy followed by many churches and teachings. A few tenets of New Thought, according to Charles S. Braden's classic history of New Thought teachings, *Spirits in Rebellion*, are as follows:

- All primary causes are internal forces.
- Mind is primary and causative.
- Man is a living soul, a child of God, a spiritual citizen in a divine universe.
- The remedy for all defect and disorder is metaphysical, in the realm of mental and spiritual causes.
- God is immanent, indwelling Spirit, all-wisdom, all-goodness, ever-present in the universe.
- Evil has no place in the world as a permanent reality; it is the absence of good.
- There is a divine humanity and a human brotherhood.
- There is present and progressive revelation.
- There is no formal creed.
- Death has no sting and disease has no terror, for they can be overcome.
- Life is crowned with joy, health and abundance, the rightful inheritance of every child of God.

All New Thought teachings, including Divine Revelation, subscribe to the belief that all difficulties can be healed through metaphysical remedies, such as prayer and affirmation. Spiritual Mind Treatment, in which mind is considered primary and causative, is the principal method of healing used in New Thought.

The New Thought movement began in the 1800s with Emma Curtis Hopkins, the founder of Divine Science; Mary Baker Eddy, founder of Christian Science; Phineas Quimby, miraculous healer; Charles and Myrtle Fillmore, founders of the Unity Church; and Ernest Holmes, founder of the Church of Religious Science. These luminaries discovered, through their study of world religions and practical applications of prayer methods, that they could use the power of prayer to create miraculous healings.

These pioneers in the Science of Mind formed the basis for all the motivational speakers that we hear today. They are the precursors to the entire New Age movement, the concept of positive thinking, and many of the sales training and self-hypnosis methods that are in use at this time. Great authors such as Norman Vincent Peale, Napoleon Hill, and Og Mandino sprang from the New Thought movement. It is amazing how little is known about New Thought by the general public, considering the fact that many of the most famous authors of the 20th century studied it, used it, and wrote about it.

The basic premise of scientific prayer is that perfection exists everywhere. Since Spirit is perfection, and since there's nowhere Spirit is not, whatever isn't perfect, doesn't really exist. Spiritual mind treatment recognizes the truth of "perfection everywhere now" behind illusory appearances of imperfection.

By healing, or "treating" your mind to recognize the truth, you can change the outcome of actions already set in motion by your previous mind-set. Once your mind is "treated," it accepts, in full trust, the law of grace to demonstrate (manifest) your prayer. By perceiving divine Spirit as the healer, by letting go and letting Spirit do the healing, your demonstration (manifestation of your goal) occurs. Here is what some spiritual prayer advocates have to say:

Ernest Holmes, author of *The Science of Mind,* defines prayer treatment this way: "...treatment is the time, process and method necessary to the changing of our thought. Treatment is changing the thought of negation, of doubt and fear, and causing it to perceive the ever-presence of God."[1]

Emmet Fox, author of *The Golden Key* says, "In scientific prayer it is God who works, and not you, and so your particular limitations or weaknesses are of no account in the process. You are only the channel through which the Divine action takes place, and your treatment will be just the getting of yourself out of the way. Beginners often get startling results at the first time of trying, for all that is absolutely essential is to have an open mind, and sufficient faith to try the experiment. Apart from that you may hold any views on religion, or none.

"As for the actual method of working, like all fundamental things, it is simplicity itself. All that you have to do is this: Stop thinking about the difficulty, whatever it is, and think about God instead. This is the complete rule, and if only you'll do this, the trouble, whatever it is, will presently disappear."[2]

A Nine-Part Prayer Formula

Credit must be given to the founders of New Thought for scientific prayer. This is a successful way to fulfill desires by using the following steps:

1. Resolution: Goal

State your intention or goal for the prayer, along with your full name or the name of the person you're praying for. Before deciding on a particular goal, make sure you've done the exercise on page 162 related to discovering your true desires. Otherwise you may get frustrated trying to get something you don't really want.

2. Reverence: Glorification

Come to certainty that divine Spirit is the source of your good. Identify where your good ultimately comes from. It's not from your limited ego, from your environment, or from chance. Divinity, the source of all good, grants the miracle of answered prayer. Acknowledging, revering, and glorifying Spirit brings a sense of gratitude and humility.

3. Rapport: Oneness

Come to certainty that you're one with divine Spirit. Unify with wholeness and attune to cosmic life. State that you're one with the divine and appreciate Spirit at work in your life, fulfilling your goal.

4. Receiving: Claim or Choice

Clearly and precisely state the goal you wish to attain (or better). Here you claim the goal of your prayer as something you already own, as belonging to you. Thus it becomes yours.

5. Renewal: Healing

Get in touch with and heal the blockages that prevent you from fulfilling your goal. Some of them may be: negative thoughts and feelings, influence of near and dear ones, societal beliefs and judgments, belief of undeserving, influence of astral entities, influence of your past, parents, church, teachers, and so on.

From deep within, you can receive understanding about those influences. Therefore, close your eyes, take some deep breaths, and ask. Your higher self will show you. Then make a list of whatever needs healing.

Use the prayers and affirmations in Chapter 11 to release limiting beliefs and to renew your mind to its pristine state of wholeness. Continue to speak prayers to heal these blockages until you come to *certainty* that you deserve your goal.

6. Realization: Certitude

Come to certainty that you deserve to have your goal and accept it. Since you healed whatever prevented you from that certainty, now you know, beyond a shadow of a doubt, your prayer is answered. Certainty is complete, perfect, and absolute, and leaves no room for the mind to waver.

7. Reward: Gratitude

Give thanks that your goal is fulfilled in advance. Since you assume your goal is already fulfilled, thank Spirit for that fulfillment.

8. Release: Letting Go

Give your prayer over to the divine, let go and let God. Release your goal into Spirit. This is the most important section of the prayer because at the moment of "letting go," the manifestation literally occurs by the operation of the law of grace. Why? For the same reason that the instant you let go of anything you've been struggling to attain, that's exactly when you get it.

9. Repose: Silence

Sit in quietude and let nature manifest your goal. After thoroughly letting go and giving over to Spirit, immediately close your eyes and give up completely. Do nothing, nothing, and less than nothing. Dwell in the silence and oneness of your being. Surrender to the divine in a state of inner repose. In that silence abides the fulfillment of all desires, including the one you just prayed for.

In the moment of silence, the physical demonstration occurs and creation is born. Here you feel ecstatic union with the divine; you see and feel your goal literally take form and materialize. Sit quietly in a state of complete rest. Savor this profound experience.

Although the complete study of scientific prayer is beyond the scope of this book, you can read books by Ernest Holmes, such as *The Science of Mind,* Catherine Ponder's books, such as *The Dynamic Laws of Prayer,* and books by Joseph Murphy, William Parker, or Jack Addington. Or you can read Dr. Peter V. Meyer and Ann Meyer's *Being a Christ!*

After studying some books about scientific prayer, compose prayers for yourself for goals that you wish to accomplish. Write down your prayers and then speak them aloud each day in a strong, clear voice, until you get the results. Make a regular time for prayer, either just before bed or first thing in the morning. It's a good idea to keep a notebook of all your prayer treatments and record the date that each one manifests. Send me a letter describing your prayer successes: Susan G. Shumsky, P.O. Box 7185, New York, NY 10116.

Birth of a Miracle

The secret of precipitation of desire is contained in the mysterious act of letting go and dwelling in the silence of absolute bliss consciousness. That's the moment of divine mystery of creation. It's said that for any new creation to arise, there must be a death to the old. By letting go and allowing nature bring about change, something new can be born.

The principle of release at the end of a scientific prayer, therefore, is the way nature functions. That's why the release imparts the magic of precipitation. By giving your prayer over to Spirit, you're letting nature's way create your miracle.

Scientific prayer takes you through a psychological process that transforms the way you look at your problem. No longer are you hopeless, desperate and lonely, fighting your environment. Instead you're cooperating with God in a glorious conspiracy of divine healing and spiritual awakening.

By uniting your limited ego with divine mind, you remember that you're a divine being. Spirit acts as your partner, and you stand beside Spirit to co-create your destiny. In this way you become captain, in command of your ship, while Spirit is your co-pilot, steering you safely to shore. Never are you alone again, for Spirit takes the rudder and leads you to your highest good.

You have the power to transform your life through the simple principles of scientific prayer. Heal yourself, heal others, and be free.

"If you can dream it, you can do it."
—Walt Disney

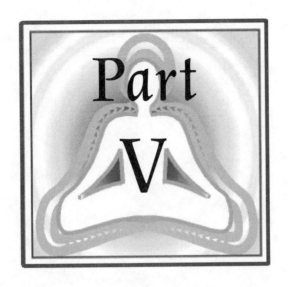

Part V

Discovering ESP

Chapter 13

pening Spiritual Sight, Sound, and Sensing

In This Chapter:
- Communicating with Spirit.
- Developing ESP.
- Following Inner Guidance.

Chapter Affirmation:
"I AM divinely inspired."

D
o you want to receive clear messages from Spirit? Do you want to communicate with the divine just like talking to a friend on the phone? It's not only possible to do this, anyone can. Contrary to what you may think, you can receive direct, divine revelations yourself, at will, anytime. Even if everything and everyone around you says you're incapable, unworthy, and undeserving to hear the "still small voice" of divine intuition, you have the power to do this right now.

We've been taught that only the "holy ones" are worthy to attain the gifts of Spirit—exalted individuals who lived at least two thousand years ago in faraway lands of legends and myths. This idea is dead wrong. This chapter rejects all such limiting beliefs about who is worthy or capable of communicating directly with Spirit.

The methods revealed here are a direct challenge to orthodoxy everywhere. My message: anyone can have direct spiritual experiences and two-way conversations with God without going through any church, scripture, pastor, or religion. What a revolution!

The Supreme Secret—Revealed!

In keeping with my insurrection, I'm going to reveal the supreme secret right now: *How you can contact and communicate with Spirit directly.*

Why guard this secret? Must we continue struggling for lifetimes, hungry for a glimpse of Spirit, practicing austerities in caves, renouncing wealth, power, and material possessions, fasting, praying, chasing cult leaders and gurus? Or can we experience Spirit right now?

Wait a minute...Perhaps I should guard the secret. Maybe I could start a religion and declare it's the only true path to God. Or, better yet, I could say no one can actually directly contact God, with one exception, of course—me.

What if I manufacture an aura of mystique around myself? I could be a mysterious personality with a special title supposedly conferred by some "high" being. I could dole out my precious wisdom crumb by crumb, charging enormous fees for each further "initiation" into "arcane mysteries."

Maybe I could be "the official emissary of Saint Germain on this planet, his only accredited channel, an alien walk-in of the 16th dimensional hierarchy from the highest vibration of the violet ray, with all of my chakras spinning on the 32nd octave of the 88th highest frequency."

Would that be impressive? I could weave such a spell of seduction with my charm and compel others to follow me.

But I know you...You're much too clever for that. You can't be fooled by subtle techniques of intrigue and psychic deception. Instead, I'll just have to reveal the supreme secret right now (which is what I wanted to do all along).

So here goes. Here's the secret. *How to experience Spirit right now*:

Just sit down. Close your eyes. Get comfortable and quiet. Take a few deep breaths. Get still. Get centered and balanced. Get into a state of inner peace and relaxation. Now just ASK.

Ask for guidance. Ask for healing, for love, for inspiration. Ask a question. Then simply wait. Within your heart an answer will come from deep inside, from the part of yourself that's connected to Spirit. You'll hear the "still small voice." The message will occur to you, just like any other thought in your mind. You'll see it, hear it, or feel it.

That's it.

Now I've done it...The sacred seal has been ripped asunder, the secret veil lifted. How to experience Spirit in one easy step: "Ask, and it shall be given unto thee."[1]

How Does the Message Come?

The answer to any question comes by asking for it. It's that simple. The trouble is we don't realize we can ask, or we don't believe we can receive, or we forget to ask. Just ask, and, according to the promise, you will receive. There's nothing you can't get. Just ask.

Once you ask, let go and let Spirit give you the answer. Don't try to hold onto the question; don't seek the answer. After you've asked, engage in the do-nothing program: Do nothing, nothing, and less than nothing. In that quiet state of mind, your answer comes.

Messages from divine Spirit appear in one of three basic ways: You might see an inner vision with your inner eye, hear an inner voice with your inner ear, or receive an inner feeling, like a gut feeling. In other words, you'll contact Spirit through one of your subtle senses.

What are "subtle senses"? Usually your senses are projected outward, toward material objects. You see, hear, feel, taste, and smell the pleasures of earthly life. However, during meditation, senses turn inward. In fact, as soon as your eyes close, your outer senses shut down and inner senses take over.

Your eyes, for example, see the outer world. But you can also "see" the inner world. Your inner eye sees with a subtle sense mechanism that usually doesn't operate in waking life. However, it's fully active at night as you dream. Through meditation the subtle senses can be developed.

Every person has one subtle sense developed more than other senses. You might naturally be more visual (seeing), more auditory (hearing), kinesthetic (feeling), gustatory (tasting), or olfactory (smelling).

How can you tell which sense predominates? For example, if you're more visual, when speaking, you'll use visual terms. You might often say, "Can't you see what I'm trying to show you?" Auditory people might say,

"Do you hear what I'm saying?" Kinesthetic people may say, "I feel that's one way to handle it." Gustatory people might say, "It makes my mouth water." Olfactory people may say, "I can smell a rotten apple."

Opening Your Inner Senses

Extrasensory perception is a misnomer. Supernormal perceptions aren't actually "extrasensory," since nothing can be perceived without the senses. They are instead "subtle sensory" or "super sensory," since subtle senses are used during ESP experiences.

What's it like to use your inner senses? It's rare to see, hear, or feel ESP experiences in the environment. Most likely your intuition will appear during meditation, with eyes closed.

Your subtle sense of sight is called "clairvoyance." "Clair" is French for "clear" and "voyance" means "sight." When you open to your inner eye, you receive insight—clear inner seeing. This might be like a motion picture playing on the inner screen of your mind. Most likely subtle visions appear with eyes closed, rather than open. Here's a description of a clairvoyant vision received by one of my students from Akron, Ohio, a beautician named Sherry McConnell:

> "When I asked how to heal my relationship with my son Brad, I saw a picture of Brad, holding hands with Jesus, floating in the air, with a golden bubble of light surrounding them. The next day, Brad's attitude toward me completely changed. He now acts much more civil, even polite at times!"

Clairaudience means "clear hearing." Subtle auditory messages don't usually sound like someone speaking. More likely they sound just like other thoughts passing through your mind. Nearly all thoughts are auditory. For example, you might have the thought: "I better go to the grocery store." Whenever you're thinking words, your inner ear hears them. Jerald Kesselman, an accountant from Denver, Colorado described his clairaudient message:

> "The message came from my heart, not my head. I heard this inner voice say, 'I love you. You are my little child. Trust in me. There is nothing to fear. You have sought me for lifetimes. Now you are home again.' Then my eyes filled with tears. I've never felt so loved."

Inner gut feelings come kinesthetically through clairsentience, "clear feeling." Most likely you receive these as subtle feelings, rather than, for example, as a breeze blowing across your face. You might get a subtle sensing about which direction to take. A feeling of great love or peace may overtake you. The boundaries of your body might seem to dissolve. Here's what happened to Marilyn La Fonte, a real estate agent from New York:

> "I was stepping off the sidewalk onto the street, holding my daughter's hand. Suddenly I felt a force push me back, like an unseen hand press on my chest. I was hurled back onto the sidewalk and pulled my daughter with me. I was stunned to see a taxi speed by a few inches in front of me, in the exact spot where we had been standing. If I hadn't been pushed back, my daughter and I would have been injured, or worse."

How can you receive divine intuitive messages yourself? Ask. That's how. Ask your higher self for a message. Ask for an answer to a question. Ask for healing, for love, for inspiration. Ask to know your true purpose. "Ask, and it shall be given unto thee."

Other Ways to Get Intuition

ESP isn't the only way to receive intuitive messages. Once you've asked, your answer might come in any number of ways. For example, perhaps you didn't get your answer during meditation. Yet, after meditation, the answer might come in a most unusual or miraculous way. Here's an example from Rick Robbins, a salesman from Des Moines, Iowa:

> "I had to attend a sales meeting in New York City, but the hotels there are so expensive, and money was tight. I didn't know anyone in New York. On the plane I meditated and asked for some ideas. For the life of me, I couldn't get any answer, so I gave up. I got off the plane at La Guardia. I was walking through the terminal when I ran into a guy from college. He had moved to New York and was going away for the weekend. He invited me to stay in his apartment in his absence and gave me his keys!"

You may get your message through a flash of insight or direct cognition, as Dave Lewis, a Yoga instructor from Santa Monica, California described:

"I asked my higher self how to advertise my new business. Later that day I was driving on the freeway when it just hit me. Suddenly the whole plan appeared in my mind like a flash of lightning."

You might get your answer in a dream. A chiropractor named Heather Bernstein from Hartford, Connecticut said:

"I wanted to know whether to marry this man that I've been dating. So right before sleep I prayed for a dream about it. That night I dreamt I was in a big house in the country and had three beautiful children with this guy. I was really happy in the dream. Picket fence and all."

You may get a warning from your higher self through an uneasy feeling. Roger Halberstadt, a computer manufacturer from Menlo Park, California said:

"We were just about to sign a multi-million dollar contract to buy parts for our computers. But something about the deal had me worried. It was a gut feeling that something was wrong. So we decided to have this guy investigated by a private detective. It turned out the parts were defective, and worse, he had scammed several other companies like he was about to scam us."

Telepathic messages are quite common. Telepathy means receiving impressions from thought waves in the atmosphere. For example, Georgina Whitehouse, a mother from Charleston, South Carolina, had this experience:

"I was just about to run some errands, but something told me I'd better stick around the house for a little while longer. I just knew that phone would ring, and I was right. Within five minutes after I had that thought, my daughter Sally called to tell me she was pregnant."

By using a form of divination, such as *I Ching*, astrology, tarot, or palmistry, you could get a clear answer from Spirit safely, as long as you use the ten tests outlined in the next chapter. Patricia Steinmacher, a cashier from San Raphael, described:

"I wanted to know whether to quit my job at the health food store, so I asked the *I Ching* whether to take this new job at a bookstore. It told me, 'Those who persevere are destroyed. Misfortune.' So I didn't take the job. Amazingly, about a month later that bookstore went out of business. Thank God I asked the *I Ching.* Otherwise I'd be out of a job now."

Your answer could possibly come from a divine messenger. Curt de Groat, a psychic from Brooklyn, New York, described this amazing experience:

"I was in a car, saving a parking space for a friend and decided to spend this time praying for the world. I thought, I don't know if my prayers will do any good. But I'll pray anyway. The next day, while waiting for my boss to open the store where I worked, I decided to visualize each passerby surrounded with golden light. Suddenly I saw a homeless vagrant out of the corner of my eye. I thought he would ask for a handout, so I avoided his eyes. But the man came right up to me, looked straight into my eyes, and said, 'What you're doing with your mind is good for the world.' I was immediately filled with golden light. When I turned to look for the man, he had disappeared."

Developing ESP

The best way to develop your ESP is to use it regularly. Just like learning any other skill, you can master ESP skills by practicing. Here are some exercises to help you develop confidence in your ability to open to Spirit and receive clear messages from the "still small voice" within. These should all be done while in a meditative state. Be sure to keep taking deep breaths to stay connected to Spirit while doing these practices. Before practicing these, study ten ways to test your intuition in the next chapter.

Speaking in Spirit

During meditation, when you receive a divine intuitive message, speak that message out loud. How do you know what to say? If you're getting a vision, describe it. For example, say, "I see an egg cracking open with a chick emerging." If you're getting a feeling, describe it. Say, "Peace," or "Love," or "My body is disappearing," or whatever you're feeling. If you're getting words, say the first thing that pops into your mind, *without editing*. At first you might hear just one word. Say that word aloud. Then two words, then a whole sentence may come. This is an incredibly powerful way to develop your ESP abilities and higher consciousness.

Singing in Spirit

Ask the divine to sing through you. You may not think you can sing, but if you let Spirit do the singing through your throat, you might be surprised. Just take a big deep breath, open your mouth, and let the tones come out. At first, the tones might come just one note at a time. Trust, and let it happen.

Dancing in Spirit

Let divine Spirit dance through you. Put on music that you love. Stand up and let your body be an instrument of Spirit. No one is watching, so let it all hang out. You might become a ballerina or a banshee. No matter what, allow it to happen, as long as you stay connected to Spirit.

Writing in Spirit

Allow divine Spirit to write through your hands. You can use a pencil, a pen, or a computer. Stay in contact with Spirit and write from your soul. Beautiful poetic expressions of great genius can come from ordinary people while connected to Spirit.

Drawing, Painting, or Sculpting in Spirit

Whether or not you have any artistic ability, take out some paper and begin to draw or paint from Spirit. Or get some clay and let Spirit play. Allow your higher self to be the artist. Get your mind out of the way, along with all preconceived notions about art. Stay connected to the divine artist in your heart.

Playing Music in Spirit

If you know how to play an instrument, let the inner musician play through you. Improvisational divine music can come when you allow your hands to be led by Spirit. Divinely inspired music lifts your vibration and soothes your soul.

Spiritual Psychokinesis

"Psycho" means mind. "Kinesis" means movement. Psychokinesis is a way to move objects by mental or spiritual means. Learn to use muscle testing, pendulum, dowsing rod, L-rods, bobber, planchette, or a table to receive divine messages. This subject is beyond the scope of this book. But once you learn the basics, you can let divine Spirit answer your questions through psychokinesis. Be sure to study the ten tests in the next chapter and use them diligently.

Mirror Gazing

At night, with all the lights out, sit in a chair about three feet in front of a mirror. Stare at your forehead with steady gaze, without focusing sharply. Let your eyes relax into soft focus, like looking at a painting with embedded pictures in it. As you gaze, your mirror image might change, disappear, or black out. Other faces may superimpose over it. You may see lights or an aura. This exercise can help you develop outer clairvoyant sight.

Psychometry

Ask for an object that someone is wearing, such as a watch. Hold it in your non-dominant hand while in a meditative state. Ask your higher self to give you impressions, feelings, or a message about the person who wears this object. This will help you develop clairvoyance, clairaudience, and clairsentience.

Why Follow Inner Guidance?

You might think it's cool to get inner guidance and then be led by Spirit every day. What a great way to live! All my problems will be solved. Life will be easy and I'll be cruisin'.

...Think again.

The only drawback to asking questions of Spirit is—You'll get the answers! If you don't want to hear the answers, this can be a problem. Following inner guidance means listening to the "still small voice" and following the wisdom it gives you.

It's easy to communicate with Spirit. We learned how to do that by asking for it. It's also easy to figure out whether the message is clear. We'll learn that in the next chapter. The hard part is trusting what you get and then actually following the guidance!

This is challenging because your higher self wants you to evolve as quickly as possible. For that to happen, you have to step out of your comfort zone and stretch the edge of your envelope. If you're willing, your higher self will give you assignments that stretch you to the max.

Following inner guidance is like jumping off cliffs. You have to trust that God will catch you—or else learn how to fly quickly. This can be the greatest adventure of your life, or the most difficult. With trust in Spirit and a little chutzpah, your life can be one of great power, energy, magnificence, and glory. You just need the faith to follow your inner guidance, with Spirit as your in-house counselor.

"The heart sees better than the eye."
—Hebrew proverb

Chapter 14

rusting Your In-house Counselor

In This Chapter:

- Recognizing the True Voice of Spirit.
- Becoming Spiritually Street-Smart.
- 10 Ways to Test Your Intuition.

Chapter Affirmation:

"I AM perfect discernment."

Have you ever become confused when trying to receive intuition? How do you know the message you're getting is the "real thing"? Can you identify "who" or "what" is giving you inner guidance?

Right now psychic development is very popular. It seems everyone declares him or herself a psychic, medium, healer, or some other "title." Many are opening to the inner planes, contacting "guides," "angels," and other "messengers." But opening indiscriminately to the inner world is as dangerous as inviting strangers into your home.

Would you open your door to a stranger? That's exactly what many people do by playing with the occult, contacting the "dead," listening to inner voices, becoming mediums, or channeling "spirit guides." You would never open your door to vagrants, so why open your awareness without identifying whom or what you're contacting?

Becoming Spiritually Street-Smart

You're street-smart when it comes to your home and property. You know how to conduct yourself on the street or subway of a big city. Now it's time to get spiritually street-smart and practice "safe spirituality" when you visit the inner realms. Know the territory by following a road map to your inner life. Attain true spiritual discernment.

Many people say, "I get intuitive messages and hear inner voices daily. I don't know who's giving me advice, but I obey it." Is this intelligent? It doesn't take a rocket scientist to determine that following the advice of unidentified voices in your mind would be confusing and dangerous. This is like being so open-minded that your brains fall out.

For example, two young girls used automatic writing to receive inner messages. One of their "spirit guides" said he was a friend of one girl's dead father and he was her "guardian angel." He told her that life didn't hold much for her and she should join him on the "other side." This little girl threw herself in front of a bus! Luckily she survived.[1]

You have within yourself all that you need. If you would trust the divine and allow Spirit to be your guide, you wouldn't seek guidance from counterfeits. There's a big difference between the true voice of Spirit and whatever else is in your mind. You can learn how to tell the difference.

This chapter helps you distinguish the inner voices and identify the source of intuitive messages. It provides 10 ways to test whether your intuition is genuine and coming from a divine source.

On Which Plane Are You a Passenger?

Your inner messages (see *Figure 14a*) come from one of four basic planes of existence. The first is the true realm of Spirit. On that level, God speaks to you directly. You can contact various aspects of your higher self, hear the voices of angels, archangels, prophets, saints, deities, and other divine beings. Your beloved dearly departed relatives who've moved into the divine light might communicate with you from the spiritual plane.

The second realm is the mental world, where all past experiences are stored. There you tap into your subconscious mind or the collective unconscious—memories and societal brainwashing from parents, church, schools, peers, society, the media, and so on. These are your belief systems, which I call your "B.S." You could visit this internal "chat room" and mistake it for a divine voice. You might reread the book you read 10 years ago

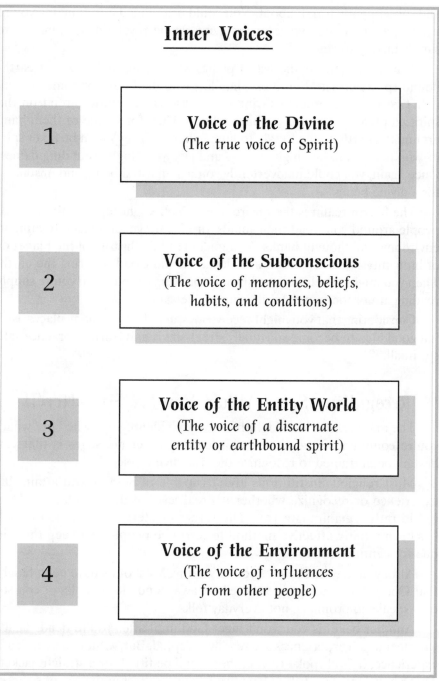

Inner Voices

1   **Voice of the Divine**
(The true voice of Spirit)

2   **Voice of the Subconscious**
(The voice of memories, beliefs,
habits, and conditions)

3   **Voice of the Entity World**
(The voice of a discarnate
entity or earthbound spirit)

4   **Voice of the Environment**
(The voice of influences
from other people)

Figure 14a.

and subsequently forgot about. You could be deluded into thinking you're hearing a true divine voice or receiving divine revelations, when you're simply talking to yourself!

The third realm is the astral plane, where you might contact earthbound spirits or astral entities—humans who died but, for some reason, didn't go into the brilliant divine light. Discarnate entities aren't on the spiritual plane, yet no longer have a body. Therefore some of them hang around the earth, trying to talk to human beings. They might be faker spirits who pretend to be "high" beings and give you "high"-sounding names. Once again, you could inadvertently contact an astral being and mistake it for a divine being.

The fourth realm is the environment. You might tap into thoughts of people around you, read their minds, or pick up general static floating in environmental thought banks. You might read the history of the planet or of humanity, which is stored in a dense mental cloud covering the earth. Then you might falsely believe Spirit is speaking to you when you're simply reading atmospheric mental flotsam and jetsam.

Considering that you might receive messages from so many places, isn't it a good idea to become spiritually street-smart and learn to practice safe spirituality?

Recognizing Spirit When You See Him/Her/It

The main reason you might have trouble identifying "who" or "what" you're communicating with when receiving inner messages is that you haven't been trained to recognize the true divine voice.

Most religious institutions aren't capable of helping you attain this experience or recognize whether it's real, even if they wanted to. They would rather manipulate you. The threat of eternal damnation in hell has been a fairly effective method to terrorize people and keep them in line for centuries.

Also, you may not believe you're worthy. Most of us have been taught that God is "out there somewhere" far away, and He (a male, of course) only speaks to prophets, not everyday folks.

Another belief is you won't meet God until after you're dead. That's why near death experiences are readily accepted. But, without a near death experience, if God spoke to you, then you'd be fitted for a straight jacket! That's how far we've drifted from true divine contact in the age of science.

It's high time to rediscover our lost ability to receive messages from Spirit whenever we want—*at will!* You don't have to read scriptures. You can receive clear divine revelations just like the authors of the original scriptures—directly. You can listen to the divine voice right in your own home.

Just close your eyes, get quiet and still, take a few deep breaths, go within, and ask for the experience. Then let go and let Spirit speak to you.

10 Ways to Test Your Intuition

Let's learn how to practice safe spirituality right now. I propose 10 basic ways to distinguish between the true voice of Spirit and "other voices" in your mind. These 10 tests help you receive divine messages clearly and precisely. You can use these to test the inner messages you're receiving, books you're reading, teachers and counselors you're visiting, and speakers you're hearing. Armed with these tests, you can't go wrong. You can study these tests in more detail in my book *Divine Revelation*.

Test 1: The Experience Test

"How does this feel?"

When you're in contact with the true realm of Spirit, you'll feel joyous, happy, protected, secure, satisfied, content, and loved. You won't be intimidated, fearful, anxious, conflicted or in doubt. You'll experience a state of oneness, wholeness, unity, and perfection. That's what the divine feels like. The experience of oneness and wholeness is the most important of the 10 tests, since it can't be faked by an astral entity.

Many people receive divine intuition but, immediately afterward, experience negative emotions as a reaction. This common experience indicates the person contacted Spirit, but then confusion, doubt, fear, and other mental negations jumped in to deny the true divine experience.

One example of being connected with Spirit while not feeling a sense of peace is a time of real danger. Then Spirit uses a more urgent vehicle—fear. A true experience of fear energizes your body to react in survival mode, a divine instinct that can save your life. Anyone who's been in mortal danger knows exactly what I'm describing. Another example is when Spirit gives you a warning signal of immanent threat. you may sense this as a bad feelng in your gut.

10 Ways to Test Your Intuition

Test 1: (The Experience)

Test 2: (The Inner Knowingness)

Test 3: (The Challenge)

Test 4: (The Name)

Test 5: (The Signal)

Test 6: (The Permission)

Test 7: (The Awareness)

Test 8: (The Quality of the Voice)

Test 9: (The Quality of the Message)

Test 10: (The Result)

Figure 14b.

Test 2: The Inner Knowingness Test

"Do I know this is true?"

You'll know that you know, beyond a shadow of doubt. You'll just *know* it. When Spirit speaks to you, you'll experience an inner certainty and conviction that's indisputable. You'll know without knowing how you know. Haven't you ever had regrets like, "I just knew I should have done that. Why didn't I listen to my intuition?" That was your inner knowing. This feeling of inner certainty isn't the same as "wishful thinking," which occurs when you want something so much that you delude yourself into thinking it's true.

Test 3: The Challenge Test

"Do you come in the name of God?"

If a stranger knocks at your door, first find out who sent him and what his business is. Similarly, if you want to receive a message, first ask the messenger, "Do you come in the name of God?" or ask, "Do you come in the name of the Christ?" If you don't get a clear, positive response, then an astral entity is present. Send that entity back to divine light by using the astral healing prayer on page 158. Then ask again, "Do you come in the name of God?" until the answer is yes.

Invariably students ask whether a faker spirit from the astral world might lie in answer to this question. Thus far, I've never experienced faker spirits lying if the question is worded as recommended. Instead they simply refuse to answer the question. In this case, immediately do the astral healing.

Some teachers suggest asking, "Do you come in the light?" I don't recommend this question. Which light are you speaking about? The 10-watt light bulb or florescent light? The light of burning hell? Bud Light?

Test 4: The Name Test

"What is your name?"

When strangers come to your door, get their calling card before letting them in. Every divine being has a name, and you can ask for it. Even God has a name. God's name is "GOD." Every aspect of your higher self and every deity, ascended or angelic being has a name. Don't be deceived, however. Beware of faker spirits who try to mislead you by giving you high-sounding false names. And don't be impressed by any entity refusing to give you a name. Instead, send that faker spirit back to the divine light by using the astral healing prayer on page 158.

Test 5: The Signal Test

"Give me your signal."

Have you ever felt touched by Spirit? Perhaps you visited an art museum and a particular painting stirred your soul. Maybe at a concert you were particularly moved by a piece of music. Or you were helping a person in need or volunteering at a hospice. Or a beautiful sunset, an inspiring movie, or a church service moved you. At the peak point of such stirring experiences, you felt goose bumps, tingling, or an energy rush. Your hair stood on end. Such a feeling is one of your divine vibrational signals.

A signal is a sign that you're in contact with a particular aspect of Spirit. Each inner name has a signal associated with it. The signal comes as a vision, sound, taste, feeling, fragrance, or body movement. For instance, Mother Mary might come to you as a vision of a pink light in your heart. To another person, Mary might give a feeling of heat in the hands. Someone else might experience Mary as a sound of celestial harps. Whenever you're in contact with Mary, you'll experience her signal. Similarly, every divine being that you contact will give you a definite sign. Whenever you're receiving clear divine intuition, the signal will be present. When the signal is over, that indicates the message is also over.

If you receive a vibrational signal, ask for the name. If you get the name, ask for the signal. Once you get the name and signal, ask for the message. "Ask, and it shall be given unto you." See page 77 for a description of some of the types of signals you might get.

Test 6: The Permission Test

"Do I have permission to ask this question?"

Before asking a particular question of your higher self, first inquire:
1.   Is it highest wisdom for me to ask this question?
     Otherwise you might be seeking fortune telling, asking an unnecessary or frivolous question, or another inappropriate

question, or you're not ready to hear the answer. Maybe the wording of your question prevents your higher self from answering it. You can refer to *Divine Revelation* to learn more about wording your questions.

2. Do I have the capacity to receive a clear answer to this question? Otherwise, for example, it may be difficult to receive an insight about a quantum physics formula, if you're not a physicist. Or about how to do solve a complex mathematical problem, if you're not a mathematician.

3. Do I have permission to ask this question? Otherwise you might be prying into someone else's business or asking something that you're not supposed to know at this time.

Test 7: The Awareness Test

"Am I alert?"

You'll be conscious, awake, aware, and alert when in contact with a true divine being. You won't leave your body and let something "take-over." You won't have lapses in memory. The only time you might be unconscious while receiving a divine message is when you're asleep at night—during a dream. Leaving your body and relinquishing control, like unconscious psychic mediumship, is a dangerous practice. It breaks mind/body coordination, causes illness and early death. Unconscious mediums may try to impress you by saying, "I don't remember what happened while I was 'under.'" Please tell me, what's impressive about checking out of the human hotel, letting a completely unknown entity check in, and letting that entity use and abuse your body?

Test 8: The Quality of the Voice Test

Does the voice sound natural?

The voice you hear with your inner ear will sound like any other thought in your mind. If you speak your message aloud, it will sound normal and natural. You won't speak with a foreign or bizarre accent or use weird gestures or theatrics. Spirit speaks in your own language with your own accent. A linguist from the University of Pittsburgh, Sarah Thomason, studied eleven channelers and discovered that none of them was speaking in an accent consistent with the time and place in which the entity supposedly lived. They were all fake.

Channelers who speak in strange accents are either being deceived by faker spirits from the lower astral plane, or they're putting on a theatrical performance, or they're unconsciously manufacturing an accent due to their own self-doubt and disbelief in their ability to receive true divine revelations. We're supposed to be impressed by channelers' strange accents. Please tell me, what's impressive about weirdness? Does God need to speak in a weird accent? Or does God speak lovingly, sweetly, poetically, and simply?

Test 9: The Quality of the Message Test

Is the message of truth?

The true message from Spirit will be helpful, uplifting, healing, relevant, practical, simple, loving, inspiring, and non-judgmental.

The divine voice will never coerce or control you with such intimidating injunctions as, "If you don't follow our religion or our deity, you'll go to hell," or "Ours is the only guru and this is the only path to God." It won't threaten or judge you with statements like, "You'll be punished for your sins," or "You are subject to karmic retribution."

Divine Spirit doesn't bring gloom-and-doom prophecies written in stone. It will never tell you to harm yourself or another. The message won't induce fear, guilt, anger, depression, or other negative emotions. It won't present conditions or demands to fulfill, such as, "Only by reading the Bible will you get to heaven." Reward and punishment aren't concepts of divine truth.

Faker spirits may try to impress you with high-sounding complicated messages. Do we have such low self-esteem that we believe if we can't understand the message, then it must be "high" or "divine"? Beware of messages that contain phrases such as, "The seventh ray of the 15th hierarchy of the 19th sector of the cosmic commission in the ashtar command."

Divine Spirit will empower you to make your own decisions and be responsible for your life. It won't enslave you with flattery. Unfortunately, humans have one major failing—susceptibility to flattery. That's how faker spirits can control us and also how many gurus keep their disciples under control. Beware of messages like, "You are the chosen ones," or "You have a higher mission than others."

Test 10: The Result Test

Do I feel energized?

Immediately after receiving a true message from a divine voice, you'll feel full, happy, elated, relieved, confident, energized, and motivated. If you feel let down, empty, hollow, drained, exhausted, or tired, then your message came from the astral or mental realm. This is one of the most important tests, since the energizing feeling can't be faked by astral entities, which aren't on the divine level.

Be aware that your subconscious mind might jump in soon after receiving a true divine message and object to the message or negate the entire experience. This simply indicates you've lost your inner divine contact and degraded to a lower realm. Don't deny or negate your divine experience.

If you're a psychic, counselor, or hands-on healer, you should feel more energized as your day unfolds. If you feel drained, it's a sure sign you're using your ego energy instead of divine energy to heal others. Let go and let Spirit do the work through you.

How to Use the 10 Tests

Be sure your inner message passes all 10 tests. One test isn't enough. I recommend that all 10 be passed to be sure you're in contact with a divine voice and not other voices. It only takes about eight seconds to use the 10 tests. Yes, you read that right. EIGHT SECONDS. The only thing that takes time is asking, "Do you come in the name of God?" "What is your name?" "Give me your signal," and "Do I have permission to ask this?" All the other tests are immediate and automatic.

> *"A piece of glass and a diamond are alike to the blind, just as falsehood and truth are both the same to the fool."*
> —Anonymous

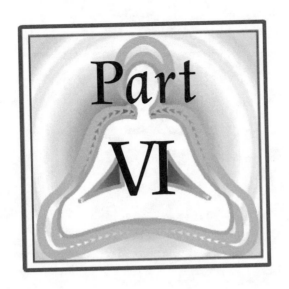

Part
VI

Discovering
Enlightenment

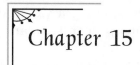

Chapter 15

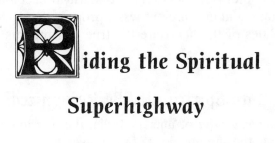

iding the Spiritual Superhighway

Chapter Affirmation:
> *"I AM the truth of being."*

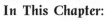

What does it mean to be spiritual? One of my students in San Diego named Gabrielle Deville was in a quandary. She believed that spirituality and marriage couldn't coexist—in order to be spiritual she must focus on God, but to be married she must focus on her mate.

I answered her this way: It's not what you *do* that makes you spiritual or non-spiritual. It's what you *are*. A worldly person with 10 children may be spiritual and a celibate person living in a cave or monastery may be unspiritual. Anyway, who's qualified to judge what's spiritual or non-spiritual?

If asked the question, "What qualities constitute a spiritual person?" how would you respond? Spiritual people are often defined as follows: practicing celibacy, feeling guilty for "sin," reading scriptures, attending religious services, denying sensory pleasures, poverty, long-suffering, hard work, sacrifice, "saving" and converting others, being a victim of persecution, fearing God, following religious precepts, wearing modest clothing, and so on.

If you notice, this list focuses on *external* activities that are interpreted as pious. These outer activities don't necessarily reflect any genuine level of spiritual attainment in consciousness. I propose that *internal* consciousness and qualities of the heart are the true constituents of a genuinely spiritual life.

Can Spirituality Be Recognized?

In the *Bhagavad Gita* of ancient India, the warrior Arjuna asks his teacher Krishna, the supreme lord of the universe:

> "O, Krishna, what is the mark of a God-realized soul, stable of mind and established in Samadhi (perfect tranquillity of mind)? How does the man of stable mind speak, how does he sit, how does he walk?"[1]

In his answer, Lord Krishna ignores how a person sits or walks, because these superficial things have nothing to do with the internal state of true spirituality. Instead he replies:

> "Arjuna, when one thoroughly abandons all cravings of the mind, and is satisfied in the self through the self, then he is called stable of mind. The sage, whose mind remains unperturbed in sorrows and pains and indifferent amidst pleasures, and who is free from passion, fear and anger, is called a sage of stable mind. He who is unattached to everything, and meeting with good and evil, neither rejoices nor recoils, who neither likes nor dislikes, his mind is stable."[2]

Thus a truly spiritual person can be described as fully satisfied, content, happy, and peaceful, without expectations, attachments, anxiety, or need. Genuine spiritual qualities are beatitudes (be-attitudes): attitudes of *being*, not *doing*. They aren't reflective of the surface level of life but instead depict traits of the heart. It's difficult to judge whether someone has imbibed such attributes, since they aren't visible. You may, however, judge your own status. If you display the following divine qualities, then you've attained higher consciousness.

True Spiritual Qualities

1. Non-judgment
2. Unconditional love
3. Trust and patience
4. Faith and conviction
5. Guilelessness and sincerity
6. Contentment
7. Inner peace
8. Serenity and tranquility
9. Joy and happiness
10. Balance and centeredness
11. Responsibility
12. Self-sufficiency and self-reliance
13. Humility
14. Flexibility
15. Non-resistance
16. Perfection
17. Compassion
18. Forgiveness
19. Purity
20. Freedom
21. Harmony
22. Divine power
23. Kindness and gentleness
24. Surrender to the divine
25. Grace
26. Spiritual maturity
27. Wisdom and enlightenment

Figure 15a.

The remainder of this chapter is devoted to understanding true spiritual qualities. Each of these qualities will be elucidated. Then scriptural references from major religions will interpret these traits.

1. Non-Judgment

Rare is the individual who judges not. For judgment is prevalent, causing conflict, strife, war, murder. Who is qualified to judge anyone? We're all divine children. No one is less or greater than another.

Scriptural References:

"The sage looks equally upon a Brahmin endowed with learning and humility, upon a cow, upon an elephant, upon a dog, and even upon a Shvapaka [the lowest caste]."[3] (Hindu).

"The souls of all people are equal, whether they live on the high mountains or at the bottoms of the valleys."[4] (Tenrikyo).

"Why beholdest thou the mote that is in thy brother's eye, but considerest not the beam that is in thine own eye?"[5] (Christian).

2. Unconditional Love

When conditions are attached to love, there is no love—only expectations. When love is given freely and fully, without strings attached, then divine love can flow. Be in love with life and with yourself, and be happy.

Scriptural References:

"Thou shalt love thy neighbor as thyself."[6] (Judeo-Christian).

"Beloved, let us love one another: for love is of God; and everyone that loveth is born of God, and knoweth God...and he that dwelleth in love dwelleth in God, and God in him."[7] (Christian).

"Those immersed in the love of God feel love for all things."[8] (Sikh).

3. Trust and Patience

Let go and let Spirit be your guide. Trust that you'll be led to your highest good. Fear not, for you are divinely protected. By giving up your agenda and following divine guidance, you'll be shown the way. Trust that divine will is at work in your life. Be patient and at peace.

Scriptural References:

"Trust in the Lord, and do good; so shalt thou dwell in the land, and verily thou shalt be fed. Delight thyself also in the Lord; and he shall give thee the desires of thine heart. Commit thy way unto the Lord; trust also in him; and he shall bring it to pass."[9] (Judeo-Christian).

"How many animals do not carry their own provision! God provides for them and for you."[10] (Islam).

"Consider the lilies of the field, how they grow; they toil not, neither do they spin: And yet I say unto you, that even Solomon in all his glory was not arrayed like one of these. Wherefore, If God so clothe the grass of the field, which today is, and tomorrow is cast into the oven, shall he not much more clothe you, O ye of little faith?"[11] (Christian).

4. Faith and Conviction

Faith brings confidence and understanding of the right path to follow. Faith gives an assured expectation of positive results and outcomes. Without faith, nothing can be accomplished. With faith, everything is possible.

Scriptural References:

"If ye have faith as a grain of mustard seed, ye shall say unto this mountain, Remove hence to yonder place; and it shall remove; and nothing shall be impossible unto you."[12] (Christian).

"And all things, whatsoever ye shall ask in prayer, believing, ye shall receive."[13] (Christian).

"One who is full of faith, is purposeful, and has mastered the senses, obtains wisdom. Having had the revelation of truth, he goes swiftly to the supreme peace. But one who lacks wisdom, without faith, with a doubting soul, goes to destruction. For the doubting soul there is neither this world, nor the world beyond, nor any happiness."[14] (Hindu).

5. Guilelessness and Sincerity

Be innocent as a little child and let go of masks and façades. Only the sincere seeker, with pure intentions, without hidden motives, can enter the divine kingdom. There's a special place in God's heart for the innocent.

Scriptural References:

"Sincerity is the single virtue that binds divinity and man in one."[15] (Shinto).

"The great man is he who does not lose his child's heart."[16] (Confucian).

"Manifest plainness, embrace simplicity, reduce selfishness, have few desires."[17] (Taoist).

6. Contentment

A contented heart, full of love, is a happy heart. The simple state of contentment is the final destination of all seekers. Contentment can't be bought in the marketplace. It can only be earned through peacefulness.

Scriptural References:

"Let your conversation be without covetousness; and be content with such things as ye have: for he hath said, I will never leave thee, nor forsake thee."[18] (Christian).

"Having abandoned attachment to actions and their fruit, always contented, dependent on nothing, seeking no refuge, one is not doing anything, though fully engaged in action. Content with whatever comes unsought, beyond the pairs of opposites, free from jealousy, balanced in success and failure, though acting one is not bound."[19] (Hindu).

"The felicity that results from the gratification of desire, or that other purer felicity which one enjoys in heaven, does not come to even a sixteenth part of that which arises upon the abandonment of all kinds of thirst!"[20] (Hindu).

7. Inner Peace

Be still and be at peace in the heart of divine love. Your inner center is the place of perfect peace, the place to return to. There you drink an infinite wellspring of peacefulness and repose.

Scriptural References:

"One attains peace into whom all desires flow as rivers flow into the ocean, which is filled with water but remains unmoved—not one who hankers after desires."[21] (Hindu).

"Thou wilt keep him in perfect peace, whose mind is stayed on thee: because he trusteth in thee."[22] (Judeo-Christian).

"If a man sings of God and hears of Him, and let love of God sprout within him, all his sorrows shall vanish, and in his mind, God will bestow abiding peace."[23] (Sikh).

8. Serenity and Tranquillity

Like the sun reflecting on a still pond, the mind in quietude knows true serenity. Your heart is at rest when your body and mind settle to silence and your breath is suspended. This evenness of mind and stillness of body is the state of *samadhi*.

Scriptural References:
"Commune with your own heart upon your bed, and be still."[24] (Judeo-Christian).

"Be still and know that I AM God."[25] (Judeo-Christian).

"Simplicity, which has no name, is free of desires. Being free of desires, it is tranquil. And the world will be at peace of its own accord."[26] (Taoist).

"Calm is his mind, calm is his speech, calm is his action, who, rightly knowing, is wholly free from defilement, perfectly peaceful and equipoised."[27] (Buddhist).

9. Joy and Happiness

Lift your heart in joy and be glad, for the divine is your indwelling Spirit, and you are one with that blessed presence each moment. Let Spirit fill you with the true joy of inner contentment. Rejoice in divine love and be happy.

Scriptural References:
"Thou wilt show me the path of life: in thy presence is fullness of joy; at thy right hand there are pleasures for evermore."[28] (Judeo-Christian).

"One who is happy within, who rejoices within, enjoying within himself the delight of the soul, who is illuminated be the inner light, such a Yogi, identified with Brahman, attains the peace of Brahman."[29] (Hindu).

"In spontaneous joy is rising the mystic melody; In the holy Word my heart feels joy and perpetually disports."[30] (Sikh).

10. Balance and Centeredness

At the center of your being is the place of perfect balance where your heart is at rest and mind is at peace. Here you find the middle way, the way of truth in centeredness, serenity, evenness, and equipoise. Be in that center of perfect equilibrium.

Scriptural References:

"I have set the Lord always before me: because he is at my right hand, I will not be shaken."[31] (Judeo-Christian).

"For one who is self-controlled and peaceful, the higher self is uniform in heat and cold, in pleasure and pain, in honor and disgrace."[32] (Hindu).

"Perform action established in divine union (Yoga), O Dhananjaya (winner of wealth), renouncing attachment and balanced evenly in success and failure; equilibrium is called Yoga."[33] (Hindu).

11. Responsibility

Responsibility is the ability to respond to any situation with equanimity. Taking responsibility means taking control of your life and not blaming others for misfortunes. Letting God be your guide is the most responsible path to follow.

Scriptural References:

"The superior man, seeing what is good, imitates it; Seeing what is bad, he corrects it in himself."[34] (Confucian).

"O ye who believe! You have charge over your own souls."[35] (Islam).

"In archery we have something resembling the Way of the superior man. When the archer misses the center of the target, he turns around and seeks for the cause of failure within himself."[36] (Confucian).

12. Self-sufficiency and Self-reliance

There's only one person you can rely on. Yourself. You're the captain of this ship. The sooner you realize this, the happier you'll be. Take command of your life, take the rudder, steer your ship on the desired course, and be free.

Scriptural References:

"If I am not for myself who is for me? And when I am for myself what am I? And if not now, when?"[37] (Jewish).

"The self is the lord of self; who else could be the lord? With self well controlled one finds a lord who is difficult to find."[38] (Buddhist).

"One who takes delight in the self alone, is satisfied in the self, is content in the self, for him verily there is nothing he need do. That great soul has no interest whatsoever for things done in this world nor for things not done; nor does he depend on any being for anything."[39] (Hindu).

13. Humility

Humility isn't self-effacement. It's self-confidence and self-reliance, the capacity to love yourself so completely that you know, beyond a shadow of doubt, that God loves you unconditionally. That's true humility.

Scriptural References:

"Except ye be converted, and become as little children, ye shall not enter the kingdom of heaven. Whosoever therefore shall humble himself as this little child, the same is greatest in the kingdom of heaven."[40] (Christian).

"He does not show himself; therefore he is luminous. He does not justify himself; therefore he becomes prominent. He does not boast of himself; therefore he is given credit. He does not brag; therefore he can endure for long. It is precisely because he does not compete that the world cannot compete with him."[41] (Taoist).

"The way of the superior man is hidden but becomes more prominent every day, whereas the way of the inferior man is conspicuous, but gradually disappears."[42] (Confucian).

14. Flexibility

If you want to know truth, give up all your opinions. If you want to know God, give up all your stubbornness. Only the malleable can be led by Spirit. Only the willing can be shown the way.

Scriptural References:

"The sage has no fixed [personal] ideas. He regards the people's ideas as his own."[43] (Taoist).

"Water sets the example for the right conduct under such circumstances. It flows on and on, and merely fills up all the places through which it flows; it does not shrink from any dangerous spot nor from any plunge, and nothing can make it lose its essential nature."[44] (Confucian).

"Take no thought for your life, what ye shall eat, or what ye shall drink; nor yet for your body, what ye shall put on. Is not the life more than meat, and the body than raiment? Take therefore no thought for the morrow: for the morrow shall take thought for the things of itself."[45] (Christian).

15. Non-Resistance

Let life flow through you like water flows downstream. Fighting gravity is a fruitless occupation. So give up the fight, let go, and let God.

Scriptural References:

"When the habit of harmlessness [ahimsa] has been attained by the yogi, in his presence no being can harbor hostility nor cause any injury."[46] (Hindu).

"Not at any time are enmities appeased here through enmity but they are appeased through non-enmity. This is the eternal law."[47] (Buddhist).

"It is impossible either to benefit him or to harm him, it is impossible either to honor him or to disgrace him. For this reason he is honored by the world."[48] (Taoist).

16. Perfection

Perfection can't be found in this world of duality. It's beyond the relative, in the plane of non-duality, oneness—the absolute. There's only one perfection, one peace, one contentment. Seek to know that, and be free.

Scriptural References:

"Every being has the Buddha Nature. This is the self."[49] (Buddhist).

"God said, Let us make man in our image, after our likeness."[50] (Judeo-Christian).

"Be ye therefore perfect, even as your Father which is in heaven is perfect."[51] (Christian).

17. Compassion

A compassionate heart, overflowing with love, judges not, but sees only truth. Compassion treats all beings as precious and all life as sacred. Empathy and heart-felt understanding arise from seeing life from the perspective of others.

Scriptural References:

"The Great Compassionate Heart is the essence of Buddhahood."[52] (Buddhist).

"One who bears no ill-will toward any being, friendly and compassionate, without attachment and egoism, balanced in pleasure and pain, forgiving, ever-content, harmonious, self-controlled, resolute, with mind and intellect dedicated to me; that devotee is dear to Me."[53] (Hindu).

"Compassion is a mind that savors only mercy and love for all sentient beings."[54] (Buddhist).

18. Forgiveness

Forgiveness is easy when you take responsibility for your own actions. Forgiveness is impossible when you blame others for your misfortunes. You're the author of your life, and others are just acting in the drama you've written.

Scriptural References:

"'Lord, how oft shall my brother sin against me, and I forgive him? till seven times?' Jesus saith unto him, 'I say not unto thee, Until seven times: but, Until seventy times seven.'"[55] (Christian).

"The best deed of a great person is to forgive and forget."[56] (Islam).

"Where there is forgiveness, there is God Himself."[57] (Sikh).

19. Purity

Purity arises from contact with the undefiled: the one wholeness, the perfection of being. At your center of being is the indwelling Spirit, where purity dwells. Purity has nothing to do with habits, lifestyle, or diet. It's reflective of consciousness at peace.

Scriptural References:

"Blessed are the pure in heart: for they shall see God."[58] (Christian).

"By purity of heart alone is the holy Eternal attained."[59] (Sikh).

"A pure heart is as a mirror; cleanse it with the burnish of love and severance from all save God, that the true sun may shine within it and the eternal morning dawn."[60] (Baha'i).

20. Freedom

Free yourself from the shackles of material world. Be in the world but not of the world. Unattached to ephemeral things, cling to the indwelling divine presence, which lasts eternally. Then you're truly free.

Scriptural References:

"When a man is free from all sense pleasures and depends on nothingness he is free in the supreme freedom from perception. He will stay there and not return again."[61] (Buddhist).

"Him I call a Brahmin who, casting off attachment to human things, rises above attachment to heavenly things, is separated from all attachments."[62] (Buddhist).

"With your mind thus established in the yoga of renunciation, you will be liberated from the bonds of karma (action), which yield good and evil fruits; freed from them, you will come unto Me."[63] (Hindu).

21. Harmony

Waves of harmony vibrate around the enlightened. Waves of discord radiate from the ignorant. Your influence can be one of harmony or discord. Choose your thoughts, words, and deeds well, and radiate peace.

Scriptural References:

"Behold, how good and how pleasant it is for brethren to dwell together in unity!"[64] (Judeo-Christian).

"Equilibrium is the great foundation of the world, and harmony its universal path. When equilibrium and harmony are realized to the highest degree, heaven and earth will attain their proper order and all things will flourish."[65] (Confucian).

"He who possesses virtue in abundance may be compared to an infant. Poisonous insects will not sting him. Fierce beasts will not seize him. Birds of prey will not strike him. His bones are weak, his sinews tender, but his grasp is firm. He does not yet know the union of male and female, but his organ is aroused. This means that his essence is at its height. He may cry all day without becoming hoarse. This means that his natural harmony is perfect. To know harmony means to be in accord with the eternal. To be in accord with the eternal means to be enlightened."[66] (Taoist).

22. Divine Power

The power of love is true power. With love as your sword and shield, no outside force can conquer you. With your mind attuned to Spirit and heart fixed in love, nothing can overpower you. You are all-powerful in divine love.

Scriptural References:

"For who is God, save the Lord? and who is a rock, save our God? God is my strength and power: and he maketh my way perfect."[67] (Judeo-Christian).

"Even the youths shall faint and be weary, and the young men shall utterly fall: But they that wait upon the Lord shall renew their strength; they shall mount up with wings as eagles; they shall run, and not be weary; and they shall walk, and not faint."[68] (Judeo-Christian).

"Be strong in the Lord, and in the power of his might....Wherefore take unto you the whole armor of God, that ye may be able to withstand in the evil day, and having done all, to stand."[69] (Christian).

23. Kindness and Gentleness

Only by being kind to yourself can you be gentle with others. Self-judgment causes harshness, while self-acceptance engenders patience. Judge not and embrace compassion. Be kind and gentle toward all beings and consider every life precious as your own.

Scriptural References:

"Blessed are the merciful: for they shall obtain mercy."[70] (Christian).

"The world stand upon three things: upon the Law, upon worship, and upon showing kindness."[71] (Jewish).

"All creatures are God's children, and those dearest to God are those who treat His children kindly."[72] (Islam).

24. Surrender to the Divine

When your heart swells with divine love, there's no thought of sacrifice or surrender; there's only the desire to serve. Love of God is total surrender. Devotion is complete freedom to live in harmony with nature, in utter happiness and contentment. Such a life is worth living, a life divine.

Scriptural References:

"I delight to do thy will, O my God: yea, thy law is within my heart."[73] (Judeo-Christian).

"Whosoever submits his will to God, while doing good, his wage is with his Lord, and no fear shall be upon him, neither shall he sorrow."[74] (Islam).

"Merge thy mind in Me, be My devotee, sacrifice to Me, prostrate thyself before Me, thou shalt come to Me. I pledge thee My troth; thou art dear to Me. Abandoning all duties come only unto Me for shelter; I will liberate you from all past sins; therefore sorrow not."[75] (Hindu).

25. Grace

Grace is harmony with nature's laws. In the right place at the right time, doing the right thing, you bask in the light of divine grace. Love is the vehicle for grace to flow into your life. Be in love with God and live in grace.

Scriptural References:

"But if ye be led of the Spirit, ye are not under the law."[76] (Christian).

"For by grace are ye saved through faith; and that not of yourselves: it is the gift of God: Not of works, lest any one should boast."[77] (Christian).

"We who live in the world, still attached to karmas, can overcome the world by thy grace alone."[78] (Hindu).

26. Spiritual Maturity

Separating wheat from chaff, knowing what's real and what's false, knowing you're in control of your destiny, willingness to guide others along the path towards freedom—that's spiritual maturity.

Scriptural References:

"Ye are the light of the world; A city that is set on a hill cannot be hid. Neither do men light a candle, and put it under a bushel, but on a candlestick; and it giveth light unto all that are in the house. Let your lights so shine before men, that they may see your good works, and glorify your Father which is in heaven."[79] (Christian).

"The scent of flowers does not travel against the wind, nor does the fragrance of sandalwood, nor of tagara or jasmine, but the fragrance of the virtuous travels even against the wind; the virtuous person pervades every direction."[80] (Buddhist).

"Good sons and daughters who accept the true Law, build the great earth, and carry the four responsibilities, become friends without being asked, for the sake of all living beings. In their great compassion, they comfort and sympathize with living beings, becoming the Dharmamother of the world."[81] (Buddhist).

27. Wisdom and Enlightenment

The transitory world of duality is a mere shadow of the brilliant divine light, the indwelling Spirit, the reality of being. Realizing who you are is the goal of human life. The enlightened see the truth, which sets them free. The ignorant mistake the phantom for reality. Truth frees you from the shackles of ignorance. Free from bondage, from the cycle of birth and death, you attain liberation.

Scriptural References:

"To know the eternal is called enlightenment. Not to know the eternal is to act blindly to result in disaster."[82] (Taoist).

"As the blazing fire turns fuel to ashes, O Arjuna, so does the fire of wisdom turn all actions into ashes. Truly there is no greater purifier in this world than wisdom; one who is perfected in yoga finds this in time within himself."[83] (Hindu).

"But those in whom ignorance is destroyed by the true wisdom of the higher self, in them, wisdom, shining like the sun, reveals the Supreme. With mind and intellect rooted in That, merged in That, established in That, solely devoted to That, their ignorance dispelled by wisdom, they attain the state from which there is no return."[84] (Hindu).

"Whatever draws the mind outward is unspiritual and whatever draws the mind inward is spiritual."
—Ramana Maharishi

Chapter 16

Guide to Mysteries

of Consciousness

In This Chapter:
- The Origins of Life.
- Discovering Your Subtle Bodies.
- Creating Your Universe.
- Seven States of Consciousness.

Chapter Affirmation:
> *"I AM Brahman."*
> —*Upanishads,* Brihad-Aranyaka
> Upanishad, 1.4.10

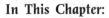hat is consciousness? Are we accidents of fate or is there a reason for us to belong to the cosmos? Where did we come from and where do we go from here? What is the ultimate reality? These are questions all seekers have asked from time immemorial. You might consider yourself powerless to answer these deep philosophical questions. But remember, you're a mighty, powerful being of pure light. All knowledge is within you. So let's see if you can come up with some answers that might satisfy you. In this chapter, we'll explore these questions.

How Did It All Begin?

Imagine an infinite wholeness without boundaries. A silent, nameless, formless void. No light, no darkness, no thought, no shape, no time, no space. How did boundaries, forms, and phenomena arise? The wisdom of ancient India offers an answer: "I am alone, may I be many." This one desire is the impetus for the universe to originate.

How does such a desire arise? By consciousness becoming aware of itself and realizing its aloneness. Brahman, becoming self-conscious, stirs, awakes, and begins to move by virtue of *maya* (that which is not, which doesn't exist).

Movement originates the universe and continues to manifest it through maya. For oneness to split into duality, maya must be the cause. That's because duality doesn't exist. Since nothing can be created from nothing, nothing was ever created. The concept that something was ever created is an illusion.

The immortal saint Dattatreya of India said, "Ether, air, fire, water and earth constitute the universe of death and birth; This is maya, the illusion, like water in a mirage. There is nothing but the pure 'I AM.'"[1]

World scriptures agree that nothing ever begins or ends:

> "All things are expressions of emptiness, not born, not destroyed."[2] (Buddhist).

> "Though unborn and immortal, the Imperishable Self, and also the Lord of all beings, yet I am born through My own Power of illusion, Maya."[3] (Hindu).

> "God, the eternally Besought of all! He neither begets nor was begotten."[4] (Islam).

> "I am the first, and I am the last; and beside me there is no God."[5] (Judeo-Christian).

Creation Is Impossible

The oldest system of Indian philosophy is the *Sankhya* system of sage Kapila. The fundamental tenant of Sankhya is that creation is impossible, because something can't come from nothing. Change implies there's something to change. Therefore, whatever is, always is, and whatever is not, never is and never has been.

Albert Einstein proposed the same idea in his theory of relativity. To him, all energy is constant; it just changes form. In fact, all the laws of physics break down at a "singularity theory" of a beginning of time, a point of infinite density and infinite curvature of space-time.

Stephen Hawking is perhaps the greatest physicist of our time, despite being paralyzed by a motor neuron disease called ALS, amyotrophic lateral sclerosis or Lou Gehrig's disease. (He currently holds the Lucasian Professorship of Mathematics at Cambridge, once held by Sir Isaac Newton and Paul Dirac.) Once the greatest advocate of "singularity" theories, in which the universe began from a singularity (big bang) and will return to a point (big crunch), now Professor Hawking seems to agree with the ancient Indian sage Kapila:

> "It may be that the universe did not really have a beginning or maybe that space-time forms a closed surface without an edge rather like the surface of the earth but in two more dimensions. If the suggestion that space-time is finite but unbounded is correct, then the 'big bang' is rather like the North Pole of the Earth. To ask what happens before the 'big bang' is rather like asking what happens on the surface of the earth one mile north of the North Pole. It's a meaningless question."[6]

What Is Life Made Of?

Please refer to the chart "Mechanics of Creation" on page 216, based on Sankhya philosophy. The sage Kapila postulates two ultimate realities, *Purusha* and *Prakriti*. These are uncaused, since causation is impossible.

Purusha is cosmic Spirit, the unevolved that doesn't evolve, the uncaused that doesn't cause anything. The absolute, ultimate reality, the knower by which all is known, the silent witness, the static background that brings continuity to creation, Purusha is like the vacuum of outer space, with no gaseous material in it and no forces acting upon it. The eternal oneness underlying the universe, it does nothing but stand in the background as a witness.

Prakriti is cosmic Substance, the unevolved that evolves. It's the uncaused that causes the phenomenal world. Prakriti, primal nature or energy, is the original substance from which all life arises, into which all returns. It doesn't create anything new but manifests what it already is. Prakriti is the creator, the silent force of nature that generates the cosmos.

Purusha and Prakriti never act independently, Purusha has no vehicle with which to act, and Prakriti has no desire to act. Only by their marriage can creation occur.

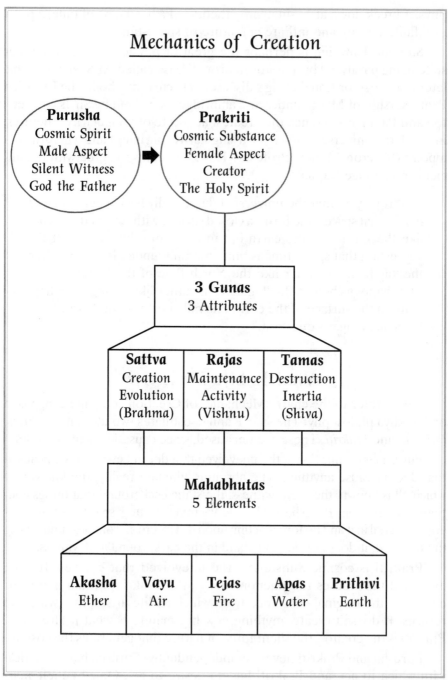

Figure 16a.

Prakriti consists of three *gunas,* attributes or modes of operation. The three gunas are *sattva:* creative aspect, *rajas:* maintaining aspect, and *tamas:* destructive aspect. Each guna has a specific function to perform, and, for life to exist, all three must act together. Nothing happens without the gunas. One force must start the movement, another force sustains it, and a third force prevents it from continuing indefinitely.

In the primordial state of Prakriti, the gunas are in perfect equilibrium, yet never merge into one. Prakriti is like a calm ocean with potential to produce waves, but silent, until a force of nature starts the waves rolling. No outside cause is needed for the first stir of activity. The inherent subtle movement of the gunas, along with Purusha's desire for creation, is enough.

When the perfect balance gets disturbed, the phenomenal world appears by virtue of the gunas. Every aspect of creation has one guna predominant and the other two subordinate. The three gunas always operate together. Never can one guna exist alone or function separately.

Please refer to the chart "Interplay of the Gunas" on page 218. During the initial spur of the gunas, rajas generates the activity to bring sattva into action. Sattva develops that activity into a new stage. Then sattva's creative motion is stopped by the inertia of tamas, which checks what's been created. Then it can develop into a new stage.

The cycle of creation, maintenance and destruction occurs by the cooperation of the gunas. Sattva and tamas govern the direction of the movement, while rajas provides energy for the movement. In short, everything in nature is born, lives, dies, and then transforms into a new state in the eternal dance of life, death, and rebirth.

The first guna, *sattva,* is the power that creates, expands, evolves, and illumines. It means "real" or "truth." Sattva focuses the mind and aids in meditation. Its presiding deity is Lord Brahma, the creator.

The second guna, *rajas,* activates the other two gunas, generates and sustains motion. It means "energy" and "action," and makes the mind wander continually. Its deity is Lord Vishnu, the preserver.

The third guna, *tamas,* is the power that stops, retards, contracts, binds, obscures, and congeals. It resists motion and produces mass, weight and inertia. It means "restraint" and "obstruction," and its deity is Lord Shiva, the destroyer.

Please refer to the chart "Vedas: Building Blocks of Creation" on page 220. According to Indian philosophy, 10 *mandalas* (circles), chapters of

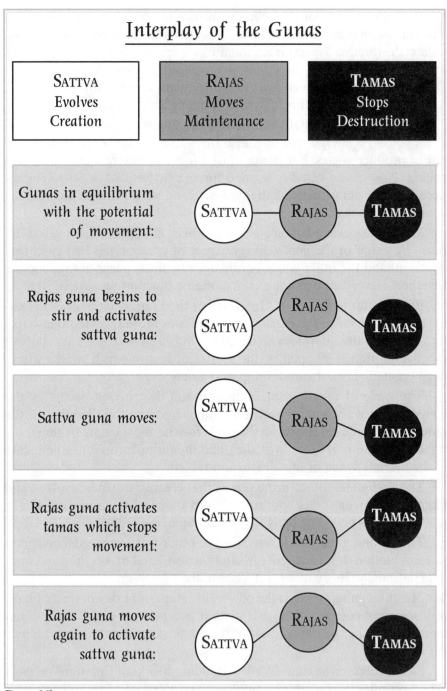

Interplay of the Gunas

| SATTVA Evolves Creation | RAJAS Moves Maintenance | TAMAS Stops Destruction |

Gunas in equilibrium with the potential of movement:

Rajas guna begins to stir and activates sattva guna:

Sattva guna moves:

Rajas guna activates tamas which stops movement:

Rajas guna moves again to activate sattva guna:

Figure 16b.

the *Vedas,* give rise to all creation. Everything in the universe, including your own body and mind, is caused by nine specific guna combinations. The 10th category, beyond the gunas, is the nameless, formless absolute.

The gunas combine as modes of psychology and bodily constitution. Your own personality will fit into one of the nine categories depicted in the chart. According to your current psycho-physiological state, which category do you fit into?

What Are We Made Of?

You aren't just a physical, material being. Your body is merely one layer of your individuality. As the apostle Paul said to the Corinthians, "There are also celestial bodies, and bodies terrestrial."[7] And, "There is a natural body, and there is a spiritual body."[8] Ernest Holmes stated, "It is our belief that we do have a body within a body to infinity."[9]

What are these other bodies and where are they located? Where do they go after death? Indeed, you have many subtle bodies that correspond to various aspects of your higher self. Your *jiva* (individuality) consists of three bodies: *stula sarira* (gross physical body), *sukshma sarira* (subtle body), and *karana sarira* (causal or seed body).

Your *stula* (gross physical body) is comprised of *annamaya kosha* (food sheath), made of elements of earth, water, fire, and space or ether. Annamaya kosha exists in *bhur loka* (physical world) and expresses existence, birth, growth, change, decay, and death.

Your *sukshma sarira* (subtle body) dwells in *bhuvar loka* (astral world) and appears as *pranamaya kosha* (vital air sheath), *manomaya kosha* (mental sheath) and *vijnanamaya kosha* (intellect sheath). Without matter, weight, or density, your subtle body is made of mind-stuff.

Pranamaya kosha (vital air sheath) is comprised of five vital airs *(pancha prana)* and five organs of action *(karma indriyas,* the power to express, procreate, excrete, grasp, and move). Known as "etheric double" or "astral body," it appears as a counterpart of the physical body and expresses hunger, thirst, heat, cold, and other physical needs.

During sleep pranamaya kosha dissociates from annamaya kosha. Sometimes it wanders in *bhuvar loka* (astral world). This is known as "astral travel," nighttime adventures that some individuals can control at will.

Vedas: Building Blocks of Creation

Guna Combinations	Qualities of Guna Combinations
1. Sattva ▪ Sattva ▪ Sattva	Purity, truth, reality, growth, evolution, tranquility, balance, attraction to Spirit, positivity, creativity, direct perception of Spirit, steady devotion to Spirit, peace, forgiveness, everlasting bliss, contentment, enlightenment, illumination, revelation.
2. Rajas ▪ Rajas ▪ Rajas	Projection, energy, action excitation, opinion, desire, defensiveness, attachment, competition, egotism, forcefulness, aggressiveness, direction argumentation, will-power, materialism.
3. Tamas ▪ Tamas ▪ Tamas	Obscuring the truth, restraint, obstruction, mass, weight, inertia, repulsion, stopping, binding, retardation, maintenance, holding fast, negativity, laziness, sleep, stupidity, unconsciousness.
4. Sattva ▪ Rajas ▪ Tamas	Absence of pride, purity, contentment, austerity, desire to study scriptures, surrender to Spirit, faith, devotion, longing for liberation, truthfulness, freshness, humility, compassion, courage, strength.
5. Sattva ▪ Tamas ▪ Rajas	Harmlessness, continence, freedom from greed, aversion to worldliness, practicing austerities, fear, nervousness, anxiety, pain, insecurity.
6. Rajas ▪ Sattva ▪ Tamas	Attachment to worldly actions, activity, intelligence, understanding, achievement, materialism, worldly power, competition, ego, willfullness.
7. Rajas ▪ Tamas ▪ Sattva	Bondage to wheel of birth and death, grief, lust, anger, greed, arrogance, jealousy, egotism, envy, revenge, hatred, criticism, falsehood, doubt, skepticism, cravings of senses.
8. Tamas ▪ Sattva ▪ Rajas	Continued subjection to wheel of birth and death, delusion, ignorance, indecision, fear, grief, pain, sadness, depression, mental illness.
9. Tamas ▪ Rajas ▪ Sattva	Vacillation of mind, ignorance, dullness delusion, stupidity, attachment to world, carelessness, lack of memory, rejection of Spirit.
10. Purusha (Beyond the 3 Gunas)	Nameless, formless, transcendental, unmanifest, absolute, unchanging, eternal, everlasting, infinite, bliss, immortal, uncreated, uncaused, unbounded, oneness, wholeness, pure consciousness, ulimited.

Figure 16c.

After death your pranamaya kosha (vital air sheath) leaves annamaya kosha (food sheath). First it hovers above the body, connected by a thin silver cord to the solar plexus, similar to an umbilical cord. When the thread breaks, the body dies. Pranamaya kosha may then appear as a ghost or spirit to friends, relatives, or those with clairvoyant sight.

Manomaya kosha (mental sheath), made of conscious mind, subconscious mind, and five senses *(jnana indriyas),* are responsible for thinking, doubt, anger, lust, exhilaration, depression, and delusion.

Vijnanamaya kosha (intellect body), consisting of intellect and ego, is a permanent vehicle that has existed since you first became a human being, millions of years ago (yes, you did read that right, *millions!*). Its functions are discrimination and decision. Whereas manamaya kosha gains knowledge through tedious logic, vijnanamaya kosha learns through intuition.

The suskshma sarira (subtle body) exists until the jiva (individual) attains *jivan mukti* (liberation of the soul). After death sukshma sarira (subtle body) first goes to bhur loka (astral plane). Then manomaya kosha (mental body) drops off, and vijnanamaya kosha (intellect body) moves onto the next plane: *swar loka* (causal world or *agni* [fire] plane), a heavenly realm.

Eventually vijnanamaya kosha retires to *mahar loka* (higher causal world) in the *karana sarira* (causal or seed body). The causal body is called *anandamaya kosha* (blissful sheath).

Why is this stuff about the subtle bodies helpful? Because it's a good idea to realize that:

- You aren't just a physical being in a physical body.
- You have an immortal soul that lasts longer than your physical body.
- There's no such thing as death.
- There's a lot more to life than meets the eye.

How Do You Fit into the Cosmos?

Please refer to a chart entitled "Constituents of Creation" on pages 222 and 223. This chart is a detailed description of creation based not only on Sankhya philosophy of sage Kapila but also ancient Yoga philosophy of sage Patanjali. Much of this chart is self-explanatory. However, let's delve more deeply into it.

Constituents of Creation

	Description	Attributes	Constituents	Functions
Body **Gross Body** (Sthula Sarira)	**Five Gross Elements** (Mahabhutas)	Gross Matter Slowed-Down Physical Objective Created by 3 Gunas	1. Ether (Akasha) 2. Air (Vayu) 3. Fire (Tejas) 4. Water (Apas) 5. Earth (Prthivi)	Constitute All Matter Last Stage of Manifestation Gross Elements of Sensation Comprise Physical World
Mind **Subtle Body** (Linga Sarira or Sukshma Sarira)	**Five Subtle Elements** (Tanmatras)	Rudiments of Matter Etherial Senses Sensed by Intuition Subtle Matter Mere Dream-Stuff	1. Sound (Sabda) 2. Touch (Sparsa) 3. Form (Rupa) 4. Flavor (Rasa) 5. Odor (Gandha)	Constitute Subtle Body Aspects of a Whole Precipitate the Elements Preceed Matter
	Sense Powers (Indriyas)	**Five Working-Senses** (Karma indriyas)	1. Express (Vak) 2. Procreate (Upastha) 3. Excrete (Payu) 4. Grasp (Pani) 5. Move (Pada)	Power of Working Ideas Power of Enjoyment Power of Rejection Power of Permeating Power of Function
		Five Knowing-Senses (Jnana indriyas)	1. Hear (Srotra) 2. Feel (Tvak) 3. See (Caksus) 4. Taste (Rasana) 5. Smell (Ghrana)	Powers of Senses Animate Sense Organs Create Pleasure and Pain Connection to Matter Receive Impressions
	Self-Awareness (Citta)	**Mind** (Manas) Conscious Mind	Cognitive Processes Conscious Activity Finite, Limited Desire, Mood, Temper Attention, Vacillation	Discovers Relationships Performs Mental Processes Rationalizes, Directs Action Perceives, Selects, Rejects Apprehends, Thinks, Ideates Imagines, Dreams, Cognizes

Constituents of Creation (Continued)

Description	Attributes	Constituents	Functions
Continued **Mind** **Subtle Body** (Linga Sarira or Sukshma Sarira)	Continued **Ego** (Ahamkara) Subconscious Mind	Instinctive Impulses Impulsive Wishing Individualized Self Pleasure and Pain	Individuating Principle Storehouse of Experiences Ego-Awareness, Identity Tests Reality
Self-Awareness (Citta)	**Intelligence** (Buddhi) Intellect Etheric-Soul Self	Direct Perception Wisdom, Knowing Non-Attachment Virtue, Memory Awareness without Ego	Intuition, Illumination Abstaction, Recognition Conceptualization Determination, Resolution Certainty, Discrimination
Cosmic Intelligence (Mahat) Great Principle Mahatattva Cosmic Will Pure Light Will of God	Has No Ideation Has No Relationship Has No Identity All-pervasive	1st Birth of Intelligence 1st Motion 1st Activity 1st Appearance 1st Product of Substance	Expands Reveals Ascertains Orders Nature's Destiny Takes a Direction
The Creator (Prakriti) The Shakti Feminine Aspect Mother of Creation Cosmic Substance Personal God Uncaused Cause Unmanifest Matter	Eternal Indestructible All-pervasive Unmanifest Primary Matter Primal Nature First Cause	3 Constituents (Gunas): 1. Creative Aspect (Sattva) 2. Maintaining Aspect (Rajas) 3. Destructive Aspect (Tamas)	Creator of Universe Primary Source of All Things Root Principle Seat of All Manifestation Cause of Phenomenal World Potential Power of Becoming Absorbs All Things
Spirit **Cosmic Body** (Karana Sarira) **The Absolute** (Purusha) The Siva Masculine Aspect Father of Creation Cosmic Spirit Soul of the Universe Impersonal God Beyond Causation	Attributeless Eternal, Changeless Indestructible All-pervasive Without Activity Static, Uncaused	Without Constituents Nameless Formless Absolute Indivisible Devoid of 3 Gunas	Animating Principle Breathes Life into Matter Source of Consciousness Directs Cosmic Evolution Brings Order to Cosmos Silent Witness of Nature

Figure 16d.

From universal *Purusha* and *Prakriti,* individuals manifest as *jiva.* The vehicle of jiva is *linga* or *sukshma sarira* (subtle body), made of 18 components: intelligence *(buddhi),* ego *(ahamkara),* mind *(manas),* five knowing-senses *(jnana indriyas),* five working-senses *(karma indriyas)* and five subtle elements *(tanmatras).* Your physical body is *sthula sarira,* material and perishable, created at birth and destroyed at death, consisting of five elements called *mahabhutas.*

Purusha and Prakriti

Purusha and Prakriti are two aspects of the absolute responsible for creating the entire universe. Their activity is by virtue of maya or illusion. Without beginning or end, they're uncaused, unmanifest, unbounded, eternal, indestructible, all-pervasive, formless, changeless, inanimate, with no center or circumference, no activity, no attribute, no parts, no form. Purusha is the masculine aspect of the absolute and Prakriti is the feminine. As Shiva and Shakti, their interaction is depicted anthropomorphically as a sexual union.

Mahat

Mahatattva (the great principle) is also called *mahat,* cosmic intelligence. Mahat is the first desire of Purusha (will of God) to create the cosmos and therefore cause a disturbance in the perfect equilibrium of the unmanifest gunas. Mahat is like a wave on a silent ocean beginning to swell. The previously undifferentiated energy of Prakriti (nature) takes a direction by virtue of mahat activating the gunas. When sattva guna first arises, it manifests as pure light. Therefore mahat is the realm of light, and from light the world is made manifest. "And God said, Let there be light; and there was light."[10]

Citta

Citta is your awareness, which can know and influence your environment. Three aspects of citta interact to cause action in your life:

1. Buddhi, which decides and resolves, is intellect, the seat of discernment, intuition, and direct perception in the individual.

2. Ahamkara, which demands, is ego, the individuating principle responsible for limitation, duality, and separation. It

differentiates wholeness and identifies the unidentifiable. By virtue of ahamkara, the universal will of God (mahat) begins to act and create life. Then an observer arises—the "I" consciousness becomes self-aware. Ahamkara is like a wave that's part of the ocean but identified as a distinct wave.

3. Manas, which perceives, is the conscious mind and principle of cognition. By virtue of manas, cosmic mind begins to think and an object of observation arises. Manas is like a wave perceiving the ocean separate from itself. Manas doesn't create anything else. It sees itself as the cognizer who recognizes the "other."

Indriyas

The 10 indriyas are abstract sense-powers, inherent capacities of cosmic mind (manas) to perceive and act. The indriyas construct the world as a system of goals or objects of desire. It can't function without a physical body. Like architectural plans, the potential for building is there, but without tools, the building can't be built.

The *jnana indriyas,* five abstract knowing-senses, are the power to hear, feel, see, taste, and smell. They work through the organs of the ears, skin, eyes, tongue and nose.

The *karma indriyas,* five abstract working-senses, are the power to express, procreate, excrete, grasp, and move. Their organs of action are the voice, sex organs, anus, hands, and feet.

The power of expression means creating ideas, not just making sounds. The power of procreation means enjoying recreation, not just having sex. The power of excretion means rejecting, not just eliminating wastes. The power of grasping means accepting, not just holding physical objects. The power of movement means mental activity, not just bodily movement.

Tanmatras

The indriyas have no real existence without objects. For example, without something to hear—that is, *sound*—nothing can be heard. Therefore, *tanmatras,* objects of senses, arise to fulfill sensory desires. These rudiments of matter are sound, touch, form, flavor, and odor. At the borderline between abstract thought-stuff and material creation, they constitute the subtlest form of matter.

Five Senses and Five Elements

	Vacuity	Motion	Luminosity	Liquidity	Solidarity
Knowing-Senses (Jnana indriyas)	Hear (Srotra)	Feel (Tvak)	See (Caksus)	Taste (Rasana)	Smell (Ghrana)
Organs of Action	Ears	Skin	Eyes	Tongue	Nose
Working-Senses (Karma indriyas)	Express (Vak)	Grasp (Pani)	Move (Pada)	Procreate (Upastha)	Excrete (Payu)
Sense Organs	Voice	Hands	Feet	Genitals	Anus
Subtle Elements (Tanmatras)	Sound (Sabda)	Touch (Sparsa)	Form (Rupa)	Flavor (Rasa)	Odor (Gandha)
Gross Elements (Mahabhutas)	Ether (Akasha)	Air (Vayu)	Fire (Tejas)	Water (Apas)	Earth (Prithivi)

Figure 16e.

Mahabhutas

Mahabhutas or *bhutas,* are the five elements. In order for tanmatras to manifest, they need a vehicle. For instance, touch can't be felt without air. The five elements are vehicles through which sense objects manifest.

To understand the relationship between indriyas, tanmatras and bhutas, please refer to the chart, "Five Senses and Five Elements" on page 226. On this chart the five elements and five senses are listed in order, from most subtle to most dense:

- Hearing is related to ether *(akasha),* the principle of vacuity and the vehicle of sound. It can be heard, but can't be felt, seen, tasted, or smelled. Sound has no touch, form, flavor or odor.

- Feeling is related to air *(vayu),* the principle of motion and the vehicle of touch, so it can be felt and heard. It has touch and sound but no form, flavor or odor. It can't be seen, tasted, or smelled.

- Seeing is related to fire *(tejas),* the principle of luminosity. It's the vehicle of form and has touch and sound, so it can be seen, felt, and heard. But it has no flavor or odor; hence, it can't be tasted or smelled.

- Taste is related to water *(apas),* the principle of liquidity and the vehicle of flavor. It has form, touch, and sound, so it can be tasted, seen, felt, and heard. But it can't be smelled.

- Smell is related to earth *(prthivi),* the principle of solidarity. It's the vehicle of odor and has flavor, form, touch, and sound. It can be smelled, tasted, seen felt, and heard. The earth element is the densest, most slowed-down vibrational form.

The five elements are transformed states of Prakriti, distilled from the three gunas. Please refer to the chart "Three Gunas and Five Elements." on page 228. The element of ether is created from sattva guna, air comes from a combination of sattva and rajas, fire is made of rajas, water from rajas and tamas, and earth from tamas guna.

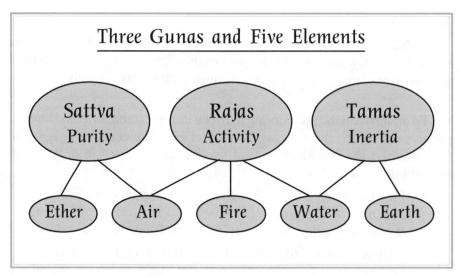

Figure 16f.

What Is Enlightenment?

The universe was created from consciousness, which underlies and vibrates through every particle of creation. Everything is made of consciousness, including you. The deep desire of every individual is to return to conscious awareness of the underlying consciousness that creates and maintains this cosmos.

Your consciousness continues intact throughout lifetimes. You've lived in many forms and might continue in many more, depending on how long you decide to hold onto your *sanskaras* (desires that have accumulated for eons). When you're ready to let go, you'll find a way out.

After lifetimes of struggle, everyone finally gives up the fight. Then that soul magnetizes to itself a path to find the way back home. The final stage of the soul's journey is to discover truth within and surrender to the divine.

Self-discovery often takes circuitous routes. But, by virtue of the fact that you're reading this book now, you're well on your way to your goal. What is the nature of the path and how will you recognize the goal?

There are seven states of consciousness you can experience. Let's discover what they are now:

1. In Deep Sleep State *(sushupti avastha)* your body is asleep and mind is unconsciousness. There are no dreams and no awareness. The EEG (brain wave patterns) shows mostly Delta activity.

2. In Dream State *(svapna avastha)* your body is asleep, but your mind is dreaming, with characteristic rapid eye movements (REM) and Theta brain activity.

3. In Waking State *(jagrat avastha)* your body and mind are alert, actively engaged in daily life. The EEG shows mostly Beta activity. Waking state is the state of ignorance.

4. In Transcendental Awareness *(turya avastha,* meaning fourth state), your mind is alert while body is quiet, yet not asleep. The body is in suspension, neither active nor inactive. The breath is neither flowing nor not flowing. The heart is neither pumping nor not pumping. The EEG shows coherent activity throughout the entire brain in Alpha band and perhaps Theta also. This is the first stage of *samadhi* that you've (hopefully) experienced while practicing meditation.

5. In Cosmic Consciousness *(turyatit chetana)* you've achieved self-realization and maintain absolute bliss consciousness permanently. Even while sleeping and dreaming, you're awake inside. All day, every day, you enjoy contentment and equanimity. Your brain activity is measured by EEG as coherent waves throughout all Delta, Theta, Alpha, and Beta bands.

    Having attained *jivan mukti* (liberation of the soul), you're no longer compelled to reincarnate. Your *sanchita karma* (big mountain of karma, see page 148) no longer exists, since your seeds of desire *(sanskaras:* storehouse of impressions) have been burnt. You've achieved *nirvana, satori,* or whatever you want to call "enlightenment," released from the wheel of birth and death. You now recognize *"Aham Brahmasmi,"* I AM that Brahman.[11]

6. In God Consciousness *(Bhagavad chetana),* you play in the lap of the divine. This is the state of complete devotion and surrender. Here you contact, experience, and communicate with God directly. Your heart and mind are fixed on the divine at all times. The channel to Spirit is fully open and developed. Here you realize, "Thou art that Brahman."

7. In Unity Consciousness, *Brahmi sthiti* or *Brahmi chetana,* no separation exists between you and God. Your heart has melted in love until the boundary has evaporated. You are one with Spirit twenty-four hours every day. Here you cognize, "I AM that Brahman. Thou art that Brahman. All this is that Brahman. That alone is." Not only do you realize your higher self is the absolute ultimate reality, but everything else is too. This entire cosmos is nothing but that same supreme reality!

Perhaps you've already had glimpses of some of these higher states of consciousness. If so, write me a letter, describe your experiences, and tell me about your progress: Susan G. Shumsky, Divine Revelation, P.O. Box 7185, New York, NY 10116, or go to my web site and send me an E-mail: http://www.divinerevelation.org.

You Are the One

Spirit isn't as far away as you may think. God isn't "out there somewhere," but deep within the fabric of your being. You are that ultimate reality. The "you" that's your true nature, your higher self, your mighty "I AM Presence," *is* the Creator.

This world, this maya, this dance of creation is your own fabrication. You desired it, asked for it, and created it. There's no one but you, and you have the ultimate power to author your life however you wish. As Jesus said, "As thou hast believed, so be it done unto thee."[12]

You're the creator of every experience, moment by moment. You might be completely unaware of how you're creating, but you're creating nevertheless, either consciously or unconsciously.

The ancient sages of India have discovered this reality. In the state of Brahman Consciousness, the end-all and be-all state of enlightenment described in Vedanta philosophy, Brahman (the absolute) is all that is and you are that Brahman.

The *Vedanta Sutras* state: "He, from whom proceeds the creation, preservation, and reconstruction of the universe, is Brahman.

"Meditation is the key to this knowledge. Without meditation, the supreme realization of your supreme self is a mere shadow. With meditation, the ultimate reality dawns—the self is all there is. I AM That. Thou art That. All this is That. That alone is. All this is Brahman *(Sarvam Khalu Idam Brahma).*"[13]

Now is the time to walk the path to supreme knowledge, and meditation is the way. Trust in Spirit to be your guide. Allow this divine presence to hold you in its loving arms and comfort you as you walk in wisdom and strength towards your goal of perfect enlightenment. Remember, your higher self is already enlightened now. Just wake up to who you really are, and recognize your beauty. Be at peace in God's love and live in God's light.

> *"We are not human beings having a spiritual experience. We are spiritual beings having a human experience."*
> —Teilhard de Chardin

pilogue

"This whole universe—from Maya down to the outward physical forms—is seen as a mere shadow of Brahman. I AM that Brahman, one without a second, subtle as ether, without beginning or end.

"I AM that Brahman, one without a second, the ground of all existences. I make all things manifest. I give form to all things. I AM within all things, yet nothing can taint me. I AM eternal, pure, unchangeable, absolute.

"I AM that Brahman, one without a second. Maya, the many-seeming, is merged in me. I AM beyond the grasp of thought, the essence of all things. I AM the truth. I AM knowledge. I AM infinite. I AM absolute bliss.

"I AM beyond action, the reality which can't change. I have neither part nor form. I AM absolute. I AM eternal. Nothing sustains me, I stand alone. I AM one without a second.

"I AM the soul of the universe. I AM all things, and above all things. I AM one without a second. I AM pure consciousness, single and universal. I AM joy. I AM life everlasting."

—Lord Shankara

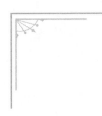

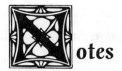otes

Chapter 2: Dialing A Direct Line to Spirit

1. Luke 17:21.
2. Exodus 3:14.
3. Genesis 1:26.

Chapter 3: A User-Friendly Guide to Your Self

1. Wachowski Brothers, The Matrix.
2. Ibid.

Chapter 4: Recharging Your Body, Mind, and Spirit

1. Anderson, *The Cultural Creatives,* pages 190-191.
2. Ibid., page 183.
3. Arberry, *The Koran,* 59.22-24.
4. Psalm 4:4.
5. Psalm 46:10.
6. Isaiah 30:15.
7. Matthew 6:6.

8. Wilson, *World Scripture,* page 314.

9. Perry, *A Treasury,* page 526.

10. Thera, *Dhammapada* 282.

11. *Bhagavad Gita,* 6.10-27.

12. Lao Tsu, *Tao Te Ching,* 10.

13. Talib, *Sri Guru Granth.* Asa Chhant, M.5, page 459.

14. Wilson, *World Scripture,* Samayika Patha, page 604.

15. Perry, *A Treasury,* Great Learning, 1, page 183.

Chapter 7: What Is Yoga?

1. *Bhagavad Gita,* 6:18-20.

2. John 1:1.

3. *Bhagavad Gita,* 2:48.

4. *Bhagavad Gita,* 2:47.

5. *Bhagavad Gita,* 2:50.

6. Lao Tsu, *Tao Te Ching.* Verse 1.

7. Satchidananda, *Yoga Sutras,* 1:3-4.

8. *Bhagavad Gita,* 4:22.

9. *Bhagavad Gita,* 2:58.

Chapter 10: Dispelling Myths about Karma

1. Galatians 6:7.

2. Luke 6:31, Matthew 7:12.

3. Matthew 8:13.

4. Matthew 19:26.

5. Galatians 5:18.

6. Romans 6:14.

7. *Bhagavad Gita,* 4:37.

8. Matthew 9:20.

9. Matthew 19:26.

Chapter 12: Making Your Dreams Come True

1. Holmes, *The Science of Mind,* page 638.
2. Fox, *The Golden Key,* page 1.

Chapter 13: Opening Spiritual Sight, Sound, and Sensing

1. Matthew 7:7.

Chapter 14: Trusting Your In-House Counselor

1. Ebon, *The Satan Trap,* page 178.

Chapter 15: Riding the Spiritual Superhighway

1. *Bhagavad Gita,* 2:54.
2. *Bhagavad Gita,* 2:55-57.
3. *Bhagavad Gita,* 5:18.
4. Nakayama, *Ofudesaki,* 13:43-45.
5. Matthew 6:3.
6. Leviticus 19:18.
7. 1 John 4:7,16.
8. Talib, *Sri Guru Granth,* Wadhans, M.1, page 557.
9. Psalm 37:3-5.
10. Irving, *The Qur'an,* 29.60.
11. Matthew 6:28-30.
12. Matthew 17:20.
13. Matthew 21:22.
14. *Bhagavad Gita,* 4:39-40.
15. White, *World Scripture,* Takatomi Senge, page 514.
16. Legge, *Mencius,* IV.B.12.
17. Lao Tsu, *Tao Te Ching.* 19.
18. Hebrews 13:5.
19. *Bhagavad Gita,* 4:20, 22.
20. Ganguli, *Mahabharata,* Shanti Parva 177.

21. *Bhagavad Gita,* 2:70.
22. Isaiah 26:3.
23. Talib, *Sri Guru Granth.*
24. Psalm 4:4.
25. Psalm 46:10.
26. Lao Tsu, *Tao Te Ching.* 37.
27. Thera, *Dhammapada* 96.
28. Psalm 16:11.
29. *Bhagavad Gita,* 5:24.
30. Talib, *Sri Guru Granth,* Majh M.5, page 97.
31. Psalm 16:8.
32. *Bhagavad Gita,* 6:7.
33. *Bhagavad Gita,* 2:48.
34. Wilhelm, *I Ching* 42.
35. Pickthall, *Qur'an,* 5:105.
36. Chan, *Chinese Philosophy,* Doctrine of the Mean 14.
37. Herford, *Talmud,* Mishnah, Abot 1:14.
38. Chan, *Chinese Philosophy,* Dhammapada 160.
39. *Bhagavad Gita,* 3:17-18.
40. Matthew 18:3-4.
41. Lao Tsu, *Tao Te Ching.* 22.
42. Chan, *Chinese Philosophy,* Doctrine of the Mean 33.
43. Lao Tsu, *Tao Te Ching.* 49.
44. Wilhelm, *I Ching* 29.
45. Matthew 6:25, 34.
46. Satchidananda, *Yoga Sutras,* 2:35.
47. Chan, *Chinese Philosophy,* Dhammapada 5.
48. Lao Tsu, *Tao Te Ching.* 56.
49. Yamamoto, *Mahaparinirvana Sutra* 214.
50. Genesis 1:26.

51. Matthew 5:48.

52. Wilson, *World Scripture*, Gandanyuha Sutra, page 87.

53. *Bhagavad Gita*, 12:13-14.

54. Nagarjuna, *Precious Garland* 437.

55. Matthew 18:21-22.

56. Wilson, *World Scripture*, Nahjul Balagha, Saying 201, page 701.

57. Talib, *Sri Guru Granth*, Shalok, Kabir, page 1372.

58. Matthew 5:8.

59. Talib, *Sri Guru Granth*, Asa-ki-Var, M.1, page 472.

60. The Seven Valleys and the Four Valleys 21.

61. Saddhatissa, *Sutta-Nipata* 1072.

62. Chan, *Chinese Philosophy*, Dhammapada 417.

63. *Bhagavad Gita*, 9:28.

64. Psalm 133:1.

65. Chan, *Chinese Philosophy*, Doctrine of the Mean 1.

66. Lao Tsu, *Tao Te Ching*. 55.

67. 2 Samuel 22:32-33.

68. Isaiah 40:30-31.

69. Ephesians 6:10, 13.

70. Matthew 5:7.

71. Herford, *Talmud*, Mishnah, Abot 1.2.

72. Wilson, *World Scripture*, Hadith of Baihaqi, page 94.

73. Psalm 40:8.

74. Arberry, *The Koran*, 2:112.

75. *Bhagavad Gita*, 18:65-66.

76. Galatians 5:18.

77. Ephesians 2:8-9.

78. Goswami, *Srimad Bhagavata Mahapurana*, 11:2.

79. Matthew 5:14-16.

80. Chan, *Chinese Philosophy,* Dhammapada 54.

81. Paul, *Buddhist Feminine,* Lion's Roar of Queen Srimala 4.

82. Lao Tsu, *Tao Te Ching,* 16.

83. *Bhagavad Gita,* 4:37-38.

84. *Bhagavad Gita,* 5:16-17.

Chapter 16: A Guide to Mysteries of Consciousness

1. Keshavadas, *Sadguru Dattatreya,* The Avaduta Gita 1:3.

2. Chan, *Chinese Philosophy,* The Heart Sutra.

3. *Bhagavad Gita,* 4:6.

4. Pickthall, *Qur'an,* 112.

5. Bible, Isaiah 44:6.

6. Ferris, *Creation of the Universe.*

7. I Corinthians 15:40.

8. I Corinthians 15:44.

9. Holmes, *The Science of Mind,* section 4, chapter 23.

10. Genesis 1:3.

11. Hume, *Upanishads,* Brihad-Aranyaka Upanishad, 1.4.10.

12. Matthew 8:13.

13. Hume, *Upanishads,* Chhandogya Upanishad, 3.14.1.

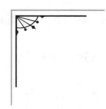

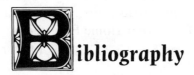

Bibliography

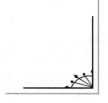

Anderson, Sherry Ruth, PhD, and Paul H. Ray, Ph.D. *The Cultural Creatives—How 50 Million People Are Changing the World.* New York: Harmony Books, 2000.

Arberry, Arthur J., trans. *The Koran Interpreted.* New York: Macmillan, 1955.

Bernard, Theos. *Hindu Philosophy.* New York: Philosophical Library, 1947.

Besant, Annie. *The Bhagavad-Gita.* Adyar, Madras, India: Theosophical Publishing House, 1973.

Braden, Charles S. *Spirits in Rebellion.* Dallas, Texas: Southern Methodist University Press, 1963.

Chaitanya, Brahmachari Ramakrishna. *For My Children, Selected Teachings of Mata Amritanandamayi.* San Ramon, California: Mata Amritanandamayi Center, 1994.

Champion, Selwyn Gurney and Dorothy Short, comps., *Readings from World Religions.* London: Watts & Co., 1951.

Chan, Wing-tsit. *A Source Book in Chinese Philosophy,* Princeton, New Jersey: Princeton University Press, 1963.

Das, Bhagavan. *The Essential Unity of All Religions.* Wheaton, Illinois: Quest Book, The Theosophical Publishing House, 1969.

Dhirendra, Brahmachari. *Yogasana Vijnana, The Science of Yoga.* India, 1966.

Ebon, Martin, ed. *The Satan Trap: Dangers of the Occult.* Garden City, New York: Doubleday and Co., Inc., 1976.

Ferris, Timothy. *The Creation of the Universe.* Northstar Associates in association with Asahi Broadcasting. Alexandria, Virginia: PBS Home Video; Atlanta, GA: Turner Home Entertainment, 1995.

Fox, Emmet. *The Golden Key.* Unity Village, Missouri: Unity School of Christianity, 1931.

Ganguli, Kisari Mohan, trans. *The Mahabharata of Krishna-Dwaipayana Vyasa.* New Delhi: Munshiram Manoharlal, 1982.

Goswami, C.L., M.A., Sastri. *Srimad Bhagavata Mahapurana.* Gorakhpur, U.P., India: Motilal Jalan, Gita Press, 1982.

Hawking, Stephen. *A Brief History of Time.* New York: Bantam Doubleday Dell, 1998.

Herford, R. Travers, Ed. *The Ethics of the Talmud: Sayings of the Fathers.* New York: Schocken Books, 1962.

Holmes, Ernest. *How to Use the Science of Mind.* New York: Dodd, Mead and Co., 1950.

Holmes, Ernest. *The Science of Mind.* New York: Dodd, Mead and Co., 1938.

Holy Bible, The. Iowa Falls, Iowa: World Bible Publishers, n.d.

Hume, R.E., trans. *The Thirteen Principal Upanishads.* Oxford: Oxford University Press, 1931.

Irving, Thomas Ballantine, trans. *The Qur'an: First American Version.* Brattleboro, Vermont: Amana Books, 1985.

Karyalaya, Gobind Bhawan. *The Bhagavadgita.* Gorakhpur, U.P. India: Gita Press, 1984.

Keshavadas, Sadguru Sant. *Sadguru Dattatreya.,* Oakland, California: Vishwa Dharma Publications, 1988.

Keyes, Ken, Jr. *Hundredth Monkey Effect.* Blue Knight Enterprises, 2000.

King, Godfre Ray. *The "I AM" Discourses.* Schaumburg, Illinois: Saint Germain Press, 1940.

Lao Tsu. Gia-Fu Feng and Jane English, trans. *Tao Te Ching.* Wildwood House, 1991.

Legge, James, trans. *The Works of Mencius.* The Chinese Classics, vol. 2. New York: Dover, 1970.

Mahesh Yogi, Maharishi. *Bhagavad Gita, a New Translation and Commentary with Sanskrit Text*. International SRM Publications, 1967.

Mahesh Yogi, Maharishi. *Science of Being and Art of Living*. New York: Signet, 1968.

Makeever, Ann Meyer. *Self-Mastery in the Christ Consciousness*. Lemon Grove, California: Dawning Publications, 1989.

Meyer, Ann P. and Peter V. Meyer. *Being a Christ!* Lemon Grove, California: Dawning Publications, 1988.

Nagarjuna. J. Hopkins and L. Rimpoche, trans. *The Precious Garland and the Song of the Four Mindfulnesses*. London: George Allen & Unwin, 1975.

Nakayama, Miki. *Ofudesaki: The Tip of the Divine Writing Brush*. Tenri City, Japan: Tenrikyo Church, 1971.

Parker, Dr. William R. and Elaine St. Johns. *Prayer Can Change Your Life*, Englewood Cliffs, New Jersey: Prentice Hall, 1957.

Paul, Diana Y. *The Buddhist Feminine Ideal*. Missoula, Montana: Scholars Press, 1980.

Pickthall, Muhammad Marmaduke, trans., *The Meaning of the Glorious Qur'an*. New York: Muslim World League, 1977.

Ponder, Catherine. *The Dynamic Laws of Prayer*, Marina del Rey, California: DeVorss & Company, 1987.

Perry, Whitall N. *A Treasury of Traditional Wisdom*. Cambridge, UK: Quinta Essentia, 1971.

Prabhavananda, Swami, and Christopher Isherwood. *Shankara's Crest Jewel of Discrimination*. Hollywood, California: Vedanta Press, 1975.

Radhakrishnan, Sarvepalli and Charles A. Moore. *A Source Book in Indian Philosophy*. Princeton, New Jersey: Princeton University Press, 1957.

Reps, Paul and Nyogen Senzaki, editor. *Zen Flesh, Zen Bones, A Collection of Zen and Pre-Zen Writings*. New York: Doubleday, 1957.

Rig-Veda Ninth Mandala. Gorkhapur, India: Gita Press, n.d.

Saddhatissa, H., trans. *The Sutta-Nipata*. London: Curzon Press: 1985.

Satchidananda, Swami. *The Yoga Sutras of Patanjali*. Buckingham, Virginia: Integral Yoga Publications, 1990.

Satyeswarananda Giri, Swami. *Babaji: The Divine Himalayan Yogi*. San Diego, California: Swami Satyeswarandanda Giri, 1984.

————. *Lahiri Mahasay: The Father of Kriya Yoga*. San Diego, California: Swami Satyeswarandanda Giri, 1983.

Scientific Research on Maharishi's Transcendental Meditation and TM-Sidhi programme: Collected Papers, Vols. 1-6. Vlodrop, Holland: Maharishi Vedic University Press.

Sheldrake, Rupert. *A New Science of Life: The Hypothesis of Morphic Resonance.* Rochester, Vermont: Inner Traditions International, 1995.

————. *The Presence of the Past: Morphic Resonance & the Habits of Nature.* Rochester, Vermont: Inner Traditions International, 1995.

Shivananda Radha, Swami. *Kundalini Yoga for the West, A Foundation for Character Building Courage and Awareness.* Spokane, Washington: Timeless Books, 1978, 1993.

Shumsky, Susan G. *Divine Revelation.* New York: Fireside, Simon & Schuster, 1996.

Svoboda, Robert E. *Aghora, At the Left Hand of God,* Albuquerque, New Mexico: Brotherhood of Life, 1986.

Talib, Gurbachan Singh, trans., *Sri Guru Granth Sahib.* Patiala, India: Publication Bureau of Punjabi University, 1984.

Tarabilda, Edward and Doug Grimes. *The Global Oracle, A Spiritual Blueprint.* Fairfield, Iowa: Sunstar Publishing, Ltd., 1997.

Thera, Narada Maha, trans., *The Dhammapada.* Colombo, Sri Lanka: Vijirarama, 1972.

Vireswarananda, Swami, and Swami Adidevananda. *Brahma-Sutras.* Mayavati, Pithoragarh, Himalayas, India: Advaita Ashrama, 1986.

Vishnu-devananda, Swami. *The Complete Illustrated Book of Yoga.* New York: Three Rivers Press, 1988.

Wachowski Brothers, The, *The Matrix,* Warner Brothers: Burbank, CA, 1999.

Wilhelm, Richard and Cary F. Baynes. *I Ching.* Princeton, New Jersey: Princeton University Press, 1950.

Wilson, Andrew, ed. International Religious Foundation. *World Scripture, A Comparative Anthology of Sacred Texts.* New York: Paragon House, 1991.

Yamamoto, Kosho, trans. *Mahaparinirvana Sutra,* 3 vols. Ube City, Japan: Karinbunko, 1973.

Yogananda, Paramahansa. *Autobiography of a Yogi*. Los Angeles: Self-Realization Fellowship, 1981.

Zubko, Andy, ed. *Treasury of Spiritual Wisdom, A Collection of 10,000 Powerful Quotations for Transforming Your Life*. San Diego: Blue Dove Press, 1996.

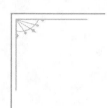

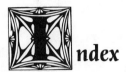ndex

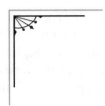

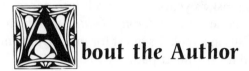bout the Author

Susan G. Shumsky, D.D. is the author of *Divine Revelation,* published by Simon & Schuster and in several foreign countries. She has practiced meditation and self-development disciplines since 1967. For seven years she resided in remote areas of the Himalayas and the Alps on the personal staff of Maharishi Mahesh Yogi, founder of Transcendental Meditation. During that time she spent many months in deep meditation and complete silence. She spent a total of 21 years living and studying in her teacher's learning institutions. Since 1985, she has studied with several other enlightened masters and teachers.

Shumsky was not born with any supernormal faculties but developed her expertise through decades of patient daily study and practice. Having walked the path herself, she can guide others along their paths.

Since 1970, she has taught meditation, self-development, and intuition to thousands of students in the United States, Canada, Europe, and the Far East. A skilled lecturer, teacher, healer, counselor, and prayer therapist, she has authored many seminars and classes and published several video and audio programs.

Dr. Shumsky received a Doctor of Divinity degree from Teaching of Intuitional Metaphysics, a New Thought teaching founded by Dr. Peter Meyer of San Diego. She is the founder of Divine Revelation, a complete technology for contacting the divine presence and listening to the inner voice. Divine Revelation is not a theoretical practice, but a proven system that has worked for thousands of students.

All of Dr. Shumsky's years of research into consciousness and inner exploration have gone into *Exploring Meditation,* which can significantly reduce many pitfalls in a seeker's quest for inner truth and greatly shorten the time required for the inner pathway to Spirit.

Since the publication of *Divine Revelation,* Dr. Shumsky has made hundreds of personal appearances and media placements. She now lives in a motor home and travels full time, presenting lectures, seminars, and media appearances, and conducting tours and retreats worldwide.

You can contact Susan G. Shumsky by calling 212-946-5132 or writing to Teaching of Intuitional Metaphysics, P.O. Box 7185, New York, NY 10116. For further information about her itinerary, Divine Revelation teachers in your area, a complete description of the Divine Revelation curriculum, to order audio and video products or to attend a retreat or a tour, check out the following web site: *www.divinerevelation.org.*